# PUMPING
# IRONY

# PUMPING IRONY

## *How to Build Muscle, Lose Weight, and Have the Last Laugh*

by Andrew Ginsburg

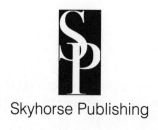

Skyhorse Publishing

Skyhorse Publishing books may be purchased in bulk at special discounts for sales promotion, corporate gifts, fund-raising, or educational purposes. Special editions can also be created to specifications. For details, contact the Special Sales Department, Skyhorse Publishing, 307 West 36th Street, 11th Floor, New York, NY 10018 or info@skyhorsepublishing.com.

Skyhorse® and Skyhorse Publishing® are registered trademarks of Skyhorse Publishing, Inc.®, a Delaware corporation.

Visit our website at www.skyhorsepublishing.com.

10 9 8 7 6 5 4 3 2 1

Library of Congress Cataloging-in-Publication Data is available on file.

Cover illustration credit Mark Collins

ISBN: 978-1-5107-1612-4
Ebook ISBN: 978-1-5107-1613-1

Printed in the United States of America

**Disclaimer: The author and publisher present this book strictly for information purposes. Be sure to consult a physician before beginning any exercise routine or dietary regimen.**

# CONTENTS

# INTRODUCTION

In *Pumping Irony*, my goal is to provide you with all of the information necessary to live a healthy lifestyle that is fun, sustainable, and maximizes your physical development. This book is broken up into two parts—the first part focuses on dispelling all of the diet and training myths that corrupt the fitness world and mapping out an easy to follow lifestyle strategy that will save you time and money, and improve your overall health. The second part of the book is prescriptive and provides you with diet strategies, workout routines, and the correct way to train your body. These tried-and-true methods have worked for over a hundred years and will be around long after the battle ropes, beach balls, and gluten-free organic kale chips have lost their appeal. The routines are designed to build lean muscle tissue that will help you burn fat by speeding up your metabolism. They are also tailored to develop proportion and symmetry so that your body is both muscular and aesthetic. Each physique is approached as an art project except that the body is the canvas, the weights the paint brush, and the food the paint. For your diet, I present you with the healthiest foods to eat, and then it is up to you to pick the ones that you enjoy most and that work for your body. Remember, you are the lab, scientist, and experiment all rolled up into one. Anybody who claims to know the perfect workout and diet for you without ever having met you is full of crap.

# PART I

# CHAPTER 1
# Caveman Craze

"If a caveman didn't eat it, neither should you," says the motto of the hugely popular (CrossFit recommended) "Paleo Diet." The only problem is that a caveman never had freshly baked bread placed in front of him or a pint of Häagen-Dazs waiting for him in the freezer. Nor did a caveman ever live past thirty.

It is important to note that none of these fad diets with catchy names are the least bit original. In the early 1900s, long before Dr. Atkins had even been born, bodybuilders and strongmen ate a high-protein, low-carb diet to facilitate muscle growth. Like a *Batman* movie remake, the names and faces keep changing, but the story remains the same—some diets tell you to cut out dairy, a few instruct you to go vegan, and a handful command you to starve yourself like it's Ramadan. Which one actually works best for your body? Even Nostradamus couldn't tell you.

For a nutrition plan to work for the long term, every individual must create his or her own specific diet to suit his or her own unique lifestyle. Feel free to name it after you because that's who it's going to work for. The idea of a total stranger creating and commanding your every meal is pure insanity. It would be like me telling you which TV shows to watch in what order—"Tomorrow, you are going to watch "Family Feud," "Law and Order," and "Wheel of Fortune." Suppose you don't like "Wheel of Fortune"? Too bad, you're watching it! If the plethora of diet books has proven anything, it's that no one diet fits all. Some people can eat carbs and lose weight while others are forced to restrict them. Some flourish on a high-fat, low-carb diet while others feel horrible and require carbs just to function. My book aims at providing an individualized plan for you. Like learning to play the guitar, I will present you with basic chords and a few simple songs, and then you get to decide whether you want to play like Eric Clapton, Jimi Hendrix, or Willie Nelson. Before we get into the prescriptive elements of the book, though, I'd like to show you that some commonly held beliefs on eating and diet are pure myth.

## SIX-MEAL FALLACY

Pick up any fitness magazine, and you will be instructed to eat six small meals a day every three hours, rather than three times a day every five. The rationale is that by consuming smaller meals more frequently, nutrients are absorbed more efficiently, and your metabolism will burn like a furnace.

Two legends of fitness past, Jack LaLanne and Bill Pearl, did not eat six meals a day but preferred a third as many, ingesting two large meals in a 24-hour cycle. They would eat their first meal after their morning workout and then have dinner in the early evening. They appeared as Greek gods, and both held the coveted Mr. America title. How is it possible that they could attain such physical perfection by eating so infrequently?

The answer can be found deep in the thirty-seven-billion-dollars-a-year supplement industry. In the very same magazines that command you to eat six times a day, supplement ads with flashy neon colors sell protein powders on virtually every other page. Now, consider the challenge of consuming six meals a day. You must eat and eat and eat, which leaves you little room to do much else. That is, of course, unless you supplement with protein shakes. So you buy the magazine, read the diet plan, buy the supplements, and everyone wins! Well, everybody except you, since you don't need six meals a day! Rather than follow a set timetable for your meals, just eat when you're hungry. Some days that may mean three meals, and others it may mean five. The key is listening and responding to your natural body rhythm. If you're not hungry for meal four of the day, don't eat it just because a magazine said you should. Instead, wait for your stomach and brain to cue you. They won't drop the ball, trust me; your head and stomach have your best intentions in mind. There is no reason to share the breastfeeding schedule of a newborn every two hours unless you are truly so hungry that you are going to cry.

I once had a friend tell me about the time she went out with a bodybuilder, and an hour into their first date, he took out a can of tuna fish and a can opener and just went to town. Can you think of anything more disgusting? Apparently, it was feeding time, and protein was his top priority. For the record, he did not get a second date.

## EAT UNTIL YOU SAY SO

You have heard it from doctors, nutritionists, and life coaches, and you've read the highbrow weight loss tip in books: Eat until you're full. That's it! That's the remedy for losing weight and then maintaining it at a healthy level. Well, it sounds easy enough, right? When your stomach no longer cries out for food, put down the fork. One concern that I have with the adage "Eat until you're full" is that it is nearly impossible to do, since it defies nature, acting as a form of sensory deprivation. That quark-sized threshold of "perfectly full" comes and goes faster than a lottery winner's earnings and ultimately leaves you "too full."

It takes about twenty minutes for the stomach to deliver the message to the brain that you in fact are full. That's about twenty minutes too late, since most of that time "on hold" is spent eating and drinking. After 200,000 years, you would think that they would have fixed this glitch in the digestive system. When you burn your finger cooking, the brain is notified immediately, and you quickly pull your hand away from the scorching pan. Clearly, the human body is more concerned with a small blister than a giant gut. To compound matters further, certain fatty foods with densely packed calories such as butter and french fries actually trick the brain into thinking that it has taken in fewer calories than it really has. Sneaky bastards!

When a plate of food is placed in front of us, the natural response is to eat all of it. This is true of dogs and humans alike. The Japanese actually adhere to the motto "hara hachi bu," which means "Eat until you are 80 percent full." Well, I am so glad that the Japanese digestive system functions with the precision of a strength tester at a county fair. Unfortunately, the American digestive system lacks that bell that rings the moment the stomach strikes 80 percent capacity. Like their cars, the Japanese stomach is clearly superior to our conventional model. Also, a high number of people who are overweight and obese have a glitch in their hormonal response known as leptin resistance. Like insulin, leptin is a hormone, and a resistance to it has been associated with type 2 diabetes and obesity.[1] Therefore, for many, eating until you're full really means eating until you're fat.

Rather than "Eat until you're full," listen to the words of the late, great Jack LaLanne, who said, "If man made it, don't eat it." By cutting out processed foods from your diet, you'll find yourself with more energy and in better shape than the guy who just eats until he's full.

## SERVING SIZES

The reason that we ignore the serving sizes listed on nutrition labels is that they are completely unrealistic. Who eats ½ cup of ice cream? A pint of ice cream is one serving, not four, according to most consumers. If you try to share a pint with three of your friends, you're either going to need another pint or you're going to need new friends. Nobody eats three Oreos, five Twizzlers, or ten M&Ms. And nobody drinks eight ounces of soda, especially when the can it comes in is twelve ounces! Also problematic is the assumption that one serving size fits all. According to the nutrition label, a 220-pound bodybuilder should be eating the same portion size as a 95-year-old, 110-pound woman. In reality, each person requires a different serving size that depends on their age, weight, body composition, and metabolism. Rather than waste ink on an arbitrary serving size that nobody will ever measure out, just tell us how many calories are in the whole damn thing. Don't tell me that there are seven servings of 190 calories in that little box of Kashi GoLean Cereal. Instead, say there are 1,330 calories in the box and allow me to work backwards. Don't worry, I'm not going to pour the whole box into a bowl; it would never fit. I'm also not going to purchase a food scale just so I can measure out 255 grams of cereal. If you look at these labels long enough, you start to wonder *Who the hell are they actually for?* They're clearly not for us, or they would be more honest with the information. It's amazing how processed food needs to be broken down into faux serving sizes while fruit comes already measured out for you. One banana, one apple, one orange, one serving.

## ORGANIC BULLSHIT

In theory, if food had its own Olympics, only organic food would be allowed to participate. All of the chicken and beef that had been injected with hormones and the apples and cucumbers covered in pesticides would be disqualified like so many athletes on the 2016 Russian Olympics team. The "organic" athletes would each be tested thoroughly to confirm that they were all in fact 95 percent free of pesticides, hormones, irradiation, and bioengineering, meeting USDA requirements. Unfortunately, the organic food industry does not operate this way and rarely monitors or tests the farming practices that produce this supposedly unblemished cuisine. In other words, organic food is bullshit, and sometimes it's even covered in fertilizer, which makes it horseshit, too.

Currently, there are an estimated 24,000 organic farms in this country and only around 80 accredited agencies to certify that the food warrants the organic seal of approval.[2] Because of the discrepancy in volume, organic food can easily be misrepresented. "Sadly, we can't trust the organic label right now," said Mischa Popoff, who used to certify organic farms. And much like the Kosher label "K" put on products, organic farmers pay the inspectors to be certified. "You're essentially paying your policing body to certify you," said Popoff. "You can see if they decertify you, well, they're not going to get their $3,000 out of you next year, and by the way, that could be $30,000 upfront. It depends on the size of your operation."

The USDA only requires certifying agents to test 5 percent of their certified operations each year, which the agents themselves get to pick. By relying on an honor system rather than rigid testing, organic producers can maximize profits by mislabeling their food. In 2012, the USDA found that 43 percent of the 571 samples of organic produce tested contained prohibited pesticide residue.[3]

Organic food typically costs 10–40 percent more than its "normal" variety, and in 2014, the organic food industry jumped 11 percent in revenue from the previous year and brought in $39 billion in the United States and $80 billion worldwide. According to a recently published TechSci report, global organic sales are forecasted to grow 16 percent by 2020.[4] Since there is no way to know if the food you are eating is truly organic, why waste your money on a hunch? You can get the same vitamins and minerals from "normal food" and have enough money left over for much more important things. So you make the decision: $10 organic apples or Netflix?

## GLUTEN

We can no longer afford to ignore how the removal of gluten from our food has caused the world around us to go straight to hell. Call me a conspiracy nut, but I believe that ISIS, global warming, school shootings, and a Donald Trump presidency are payback for the way that we have mistreated the wheat protein. Without a doubt, it is time to put the gluten back into the food and save this planet before it's too late.

Ten years ago, nobody had heard of gluten, and now it is vilified worst than Stalin. "It's making me fat! It's making me tired! It's making me sick!" Is it really? Is gluten the real reason this country is overweight? It depends on whom you ask. Since I'm writing this, I am going to tell you that this whole gluten-free craze is 100 percent Grade A, USDA-Approved, pesticide-free, grass-fed, organic bullshit. The only people who need to eliminate gluten from their diet are the 1 percent of us who suffer from celiac disease or the less than 1 percent who are gluten intolerant. Otherwise, an occasional gluten-packed meal is fine.

Now, for the love of God, what the hell is gluten? It's a protein found in wheat that gives food taste and texture. Most grains, breads, cereals, pastas, baked goods, and flour mixes are high in gluten unless otherwise labeled as gluten-free. When companies remove gluten from their products, they need to find another way to make it palatable, so they take out the gluten and replace it with sugar, salt, and fat. Some gluten-free foods have up to seven times the amount of salt as the original version, and at twice the price. So any attempt to lose weight by eating gluten-free will mean missing out on key nutrients. According to Dr. Emma Williams of the British Nutrition Foundation, "Wheat forms a staple part of the diet. Since wheat flour is found in a vast array of foods, from mustard to bread, it is a vital source of calcium, iron, Vitamin B, and fiber. Eliminating a food group can lead to plummeting energy levels and hypoglycemic headaches caused by a lack of carbohydrate.

Not only is it a waste of time and money when there's no real problem, it can make your attempts to lose weight backfire."[5]

## MEAT IS OKAY

Two million years ago, the first hominids ate crocodile, turtles, and fish to survive. They were neither vegans nor pescatarians and even ate hippopotamus, a great source of protein, complete with all nine essential amino acids. According to geologist Naomi Levin, "The wet and marshy environment gave early pre-humans a way to increase the protein in their diets and grow larger brains while possibly avoiding contact with larger carnivores, such as hyenas and lions."[6] If they had eaten a strictly vegan diet, their brains would not have grown, and they would have become extinct like the Malagasy hippopotamus, which the hominids devoured at dinner.

I have heard numerous explanations for a vegetarian lifestyle. One vegan even told me that she won't eat anything that has eyes (because if something has eyes, it has feelings). Well, I'm glad she has a good reason. I guess that means no gummy bears, no animal crackers, and no Hello Kitty cupcakes. One proud pescatarian told me that he won't eat meat because he wants to make the world a better place. That's great, but you're allowed to eat fish? If you're going to cherry-pick, you should be glad to know that the sweet fruit is high in both potassium and Vitamin C.

If nobody ate meat ever again, we would not reach a higher spiritual plane, live to be 200, or enjoy peace on Earth. Wars would still be fought, racism would endure, and Kim Kardashian would sill post nude selfies every ten seconds on Instagram. At the domestic level, we would continue to overdose on sugar and processed foods, and we would still have the same overweight neighbor seated next to us in economy. Professional athletes would be less muscular and lose speed on a plant-based diet of incomplete proteins, and Thanksgiving and Shabbat dinner would lose all appeal. And what about the poor chickens, pigs, and cows, you ask? Well, they would probably starve to death and become extinct because no farmer would raise them without the prospect of selling their meat and eggs. I don't care how much yoga you do, how much kale you eat, or how many soup kitchens you volunteer for, you are not going to open a homeless shelter for chickens. It's unrealistic (and just imagine the smell)!

Sanctimonious and hypocritical is the preachy vegan that insists one cannot lose weight, be healthy, or even act morally on a diet that includes meat. In the book *Skinny Bitch*, the authors go as far as saying, "So, yeah, if you want to get skinny, you've got to be a vegetarian—someone who doesn't

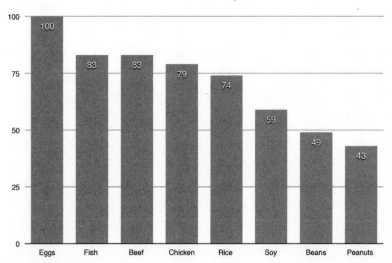

**Protein Bioavailability Chart**

eat dead animals or seafood."[7] This statement is idiotic, short-sighted, and completely false. To get "skinny" has nothing to do with being a vegetarian, just as getting fat has nothing to do with eating animals. There are millions of skinny people who eat meat and fish, just as there are a legion of overweight ones who don't. Calorie consumption, activity level, and smart food choices are what ultimately shape your body. Remember, muscles are composed of protein, and the building blocks of protein are amino acids. Chicken, fish, and eggs are complete proteins, which means that they contain all nine of the essential amino acids, while vegan favorites such as nuts, seeds, and legumes are inferior, incomplete proteins. A diet that includes complete proteins such as chicken and fish is a blueprint for getting "skinny."

Since red meat is high in saturated fat, I would limit consumption to once a week and choose lean cuts such as sirloin and top round over the fattier ribeye and T-bone. Whether you choose to eat animals or not is your own business. But vegans, I ask you to keep thy diet (much like religion) to thyself.

## GOT MILK? NOPE

Unless you are a baby calf, you should not be drinking milk from a cow. In fact, the only time that "Milk does a body good" is when that body is ten pounds and the milk shoots out of a woman's breast. Milk is a maternal lactating secretion, a short-term nutrient for babies. Other mammals like gorillas and chimpanzees only drink milk when they're a baby and never touch it again.

Most adults cannot drink milk because it makes them ill. Whether it's lactose intolerance or intestinal discomfort, the white liquid from the mammary glands can wreak havoc on the digestive system. Sure, milk goes great with cereal and mixes nicely with chocolate syrup, but as for fighting against osteoporosis, milk is pretty much useless.[8] The best way to keep bones strong is through exercise and vitamins D and K. You can consume vitamin D through sources like salmon, tuna, and eggs. Veggies like spinach, broccoli, and brussels sprouts are all good sources of vitamin K. Also, not smoking and cutting down on booze are essential for bone health. Swedish researchers found that drinking more than one glass of milk per day may double your risk of ovarian cancer, while a Harvard study found that men who consumed more than two dairy servings per day had a 34 percent increased risk of developing prostate cancer, compared with those who consumed little or no dairy.[9]

A typical Ashkenazi Jew, I am lactose intolerant and have not had milk in over fifteen years. My skin, bones, and muscles are perfectly fine with that, and I eat broccoli for calcium, salmon for Vitamin D, and spinach for riboflavin. In fact, the less dairy you consume, the better shape you will be in.

## HEALTHY EATING ON A BUDGET

In a healthy world, carrot sticks would cost less than M&Ms, skinless chicken breast would be cheaper than chicken nuggets, and Alaskan salmon would run you fewer shekels than a Big Mac. Unfortunately, we live in a government-subsidized world where processed food is cost-efficient, while healthy, wholesome cuisine can empty your wallet. Is it worth being broke to be fit? No. Is there a way around this dilemma? Yes! Get a second job, find a "sugar mama" or "sugar daddy," or buy these healthy, inexpensive foods and follow these tips:

1. **Tuna Fish** – The human cat food will run you less than two dollars a can and is packed with protein. Use

Hellmann's Light Mayo instead of regular mayo, since it has less fat and still retains the glorious taste. Consult your doctor about how much tuna fish you can consume (especially if you are pregnant), because of the high mercury level.

2. **Eggs** – A dozen eggs shouldn't run you more than three bucks and has the highest bioavailability of any protein. Try and buy eggs that are filled with essential fatty acids such as Omega-3, often labeled on the egg crate. Most important, eat the yolk. It has virtually all of the vitamins and minerals, half of the protein, and all of the taste of the egg.

3. **Oatmeal** – The magic mush costs about five dollars for a monster tub that should last you a few weeks. And by oatmeal, I don't mean Instant Oatmeal! That's loaded with sugar and hardly has any fiber. I'm talking raw oats! Add some honey to your raw oats, and you'll have more energy than a "coked up" Lawrence Taylor.

4. Don't waste money on organic food. It's a farce, and a brilliant one at that. Chances are, the apples all fell off the same tree, despite the fancy section in the supermarket. Nothing like buying a 10-dollar organic apple and then washing it off in sulfur-infested tap water.

5. **Bananas** – Cheap, radioactive (albeit slightly), and loaded with potassium, they are easy to digest, and the sugar goes right into your bloodstream. The beauty of fruit lies in quick energy.

6. When purchasing meat, buy in bulk. Buy the four-pound package of boneless, skinless chicken breasts over the organic, farm-raised, rabbi-blessed, glatt kosher, over-salted, carefully trimmed one-pound rip-off.

7. Cook more, eat out less. Nothing will empty your wallet faster than the $35 Atlantic salmon you could have prepared for eight bucks in your kitchen.
8. Go easy on the sushi. The over-priced art project on the wooden block with pretty colors will leave you living out of a dumpster.
9. Buy the $12 bottle of red wine over the $85 one. This one is self-explanatory.
10. Make your own protein shakes. I use Isopure whey protein, and each shake comes out to about 3 dollars versus the $10 version at juice bars.

## PORTLY PITFALLS

Most unfortunate is when people believe that they are eating healthy and then watch the numbers on the scale skyrocket. "All I had was a bran muffin! How the hell am I two pounds heavier?" Here are some "healthy foods" that will pack on the poundage in no time:

1. **Dried fruits:** A cup of grapes is 60 calories, while a cup of raisins in 460. Yes, nature's candy creates nature's flab.
2. **Granola:** Usually served with yogurt, these clustered nuts are loaded with sugar. Do yourself a favor and eat oatmeal instead.
3. **Bran Muffins:** At 500 calories a muffin, you might as well add vanilla icing and turn it into a cupcake.
4. **Diet Microwave Dinners:** What they remove in fat and calories, they replace with salt. Unless you enjoy being bloated, keep these out of the freezer.
5. **Nuts:** Whether they are almonds, cashews, peanuts, or walnuts, they are high in fat and extremely caloric. One handful is healthy, while two or three is a disaster.

6. **Frozen Yogurt:** Though yogurt sounds healthy, this frozen dessert contains more than just milk and bacteria. Add in artificial sweeteners, flavors, and coloring, and you have yourself a tart version of ice cream at twice the price. They shouldn't refer to it as froyo, they should call it "toppings." The yogurt merely serves as a bed of lettuce to cover with layers of Reese's Peanut Butter Cups, cookie dough, chocolate chips, and coconut. The yogurt itself is bland and boring, and even the self-serve yogurt lever is just slightly more interesting than pumping a ketchup dispenser. The goal is to move quickly past the yogurt portion of the show to the candy store that lies ahead. Unless it's your cheat day (see page 26), stay away from froyo, I mean toppings.

---

### TAKEAWAYS

- Listen to your body and only eat when you're hungry. Let your natural body rhythm define when and how much you eat.
- Don't waste your money on organic food. It's a total farce. Buy normal food that won't empty your wallet.
- Ignore the serving sizes on nutrition labels. They assume a one-size-fits-all serving size, which is useless.
- Enjoy chicken and fish and ignore the preachy vegan with the messianic complex.
- Eat as little dairy as possible.
- Buy healthy food in bulk such as chicken breasts, eggs, fruits, and vegetables.

# CHAPTER 2
# Diet Starts Tomorrow

"Diet starts tomorrow." "Tomorrow I'm working out for five hours and eating nothing but salad." "After tonight, I'm never ever drinking again." We have all made these empty declarations after a gluttonous meal, and they are all born out of guilt. There's Jewish guilt, Catholic guilt, infantile guilt, parental guilt, shadow guilt, guilt for inactivity, and by far the most common, guilt for activity. Though stressful, guilt can actually motivate and is a healthy emotion (to an extent) that everyone short of serial killers and their defense lawyers experience. But what fun is eating pizza and ice cream if the voice in your head is pummeling you as you chew it? And even less enjoyable is dining with a person who must vocalize their guilt and comment on all the of the calories that they are ingesting. "Oh my God, this cake is so rich. It's probably like a thousand calories," as if everyone else at the table thought it was health food. At the dinner table, do everybody a favor and keep your guilt to yourself. The truth is that no one meal is going to make you fat. If you pig out one day, don't do it the next. In fact, plan that "cheat day" in advance and enjoy the hell out of it! A professional tennis player puts the last point he played out of his mind because he knows that it will be of no help with the next one. If he buries an easy overhead into the bottom of the net and then dwells on the missed shot, there's a good chance he'll lose the next point followed by the game, set, and finally the match.

Far worse than guilt is the shame that some people feel after they stray from their diet in a moment of weakness. To be clear, author Brene Brown defines the two emotions in her book *Daring Greatly* as the following: "Guilt is saying 'I did something bad' while shame insists 'I am bad.'"[1] When you eat five slices of a pizza for lunch instead of the salad that you had originally planned on, guilt says, "I shouldn't have done that," while shame shouts out, "I suck, I'm garbage, why do I even try?" Being a good person who feels worthy of love and offers love is far more important than having a nice butt and a tight stomach. Of course, if you can have it all, that would be ideal, and it is my goal to help you achieve that.

When you choose to live a healthy lifestyle and eat nutrient-dense foods, you will have some friends who support your decision and others who are just downright hostile. At dinner, when you don't order an appetizer or you say no to dessert, they'll heckle you incessantly: "You're no fun. How can you just eat a salad with grilled chicken? I'd get so bored if I ate like that." Of course, they say this after eating two baskets of bread, three appetizers, a 12-ounce steak, and a giant piece of cake. The reason why they choose to berate you is less important than how you respond. Their comments may be rooted in anger, envy, jealousy, or a combination of the three. Some may assume that you're judging their unhealthy eating, while others don't want to see their funny, fat friend become less fat and funny. When people criticize your healthy eating, repeat back to them exactly what they said, "That's true, one cookie won't kill me. And you're right, I'm no fun." Or just confront them and say, "I'm just trying to eat healthy, so stop giving me shit." Like a recovering alcoholic, don't fall off the wagon on someone else's account. And if you have trouble handling people like this, avoid them like the plague.

A few nights ago, I had dinner with my two sisters and ate enough sushi to fill the Atlantic Ocean seven times over. After dinner, I was not satisfied and opted for dessert. But not just any dessert! No, I wanted two chocolate chip walnut cookies from Levain Bakery (if you've never had them, you have not lived a full life). Located on West 74th Street in Manhattan, Levain consistently boasts an average line that extends down an entire block. Each cookie is the size of a hockey puck, costs four bucks, and is probably close to one thousand calories. My older sister had a small piece, and then I devoured the rest. After my bag was empty and my face and fingers covered in chocolate, my sister asked me if I was going to feel guilty later for having them. I said, "Nope." She said, "Not at all, not even a little?" I said "No, I'd feel guilty if I didn't have them." I wanted them, I planned on having them, and I deserved them. This was my day to splurge, and I stuck to the script. In other words, "Diet starts tomorrow."

## DINNER

Life in the United States is based around dinner. What's for dinner? Where are we going for dinner? Want to grab dinner? Unfortunately, "going out to eat" usually means "going out to get fat." You have a few of glasses of wine, some bread to go with your fried calamari, followed by a porterhouse steak and chocolate mousse cake. Not only do you feel sick after this splurge, but you wake up the next morning with a new paunch. By contrast, in Italy, instead of dinner, lunch is their main event, and amazingly, fewer people in Italy are fat! How is this possible? Well, we eat larger portions, more processed foods with higher fat, and average 2,700 calories a day.[2] The problem is that the average person only burns around 2,000 calories, thereby leaving a 700-calorie surplus. A pound of body fat can be gained by eating an excess of 3,500 calories. So, five days at a 700-calorie surplus and voilà, your ass has grown to the size of a bowling ball. Divide 365 days by 5, and you have gained 73 pounds in a year! Hospital bed, here we come!

Blind dates, client meetings, and hanging out with friends will land you in a restaurant that prides itself on filling you up with food and booze until the check is fat and your stomach is about to explode. Here's how to counter the waiter who makes his sales pitch with words like "caramelized," "classic," "crunchy," "creamy," "glazed," "hearty," "homemade," "infused," "pickled," "poached," "pureed," "sautéed," "seared," "simmered," "smoked," "smothered," "sweet," "tender," "velvety," and "zesty." Allow the waiter to perform his monologue, and then order what you had planned on before dinner. That's right, go online, look at the menu, and pick your entrée and appetizers ahead of time.

During the course of the meal, you will be handed up to three menus: a wine list, a main menu of appetizers and entrées, and finally, one for dessert. Each piece of literature is distinct in its size, font, and overall layout. The wine list may resemble a leather-bound copy of *The Iliad*, while the dessert menu will have the boldest, most luxuriant print on the smallest sheet of paper. All of this paperwork unconsciously causes us to order more food, since it's harder to say no to dessert when the choices are lavishly printed on the likes of a wedding invitation. Unless it's a birthday or anniversary celebration, don't give in. If you're invited for an after-dinner drink, say, "No, thanks." Your stomach is full enough!

## THE EARLY BIRD SPECIAL

When I was a kid, my family woke up at 5:30 in the morning and went to bed at 9:30 at night. Dinner at the Ginsburg house was usually served around 5:30 p.m., while dinner at a friend's house was much later than I was used to. Some families ate at 6:30, others dined at 7, and some even broke bread at 8!

As an adult, I still adhere to an "early" schedule. I wake up at 5:20 a.m., eat breakfast at 5:40, and tend to eat dinner around 6 p.m. In New York City, a 6 p.m. dinner is a subject of ridicule, and a 10 p.m. bedtime is unheard of. Luckily, I gave up trying to be trendy a long time ago. I'm not waiting until 8 p.m. to eat dinner like the cool kids or go to bed at 2 a.m. like the barfly. To maximize digestion and quality of sleep, one should eat dinner at least three hours before going to bed. The closer you eat to bedtime, the higher your blood sugar and insulin will spike, and the harder it will be for you to fall asleep. So go ahead and make fun of me. Say, "You and my grandma should catch the early bird special sometime." Yes, we probably should. Give me her number, and we'll set that up.

## DON'T BRING IT HOME

Whether it's a pint of Ben and Jerry's, a block of cheese, or pneumonia, just don't bring it home. I know that if there is a pint of ice cream sitting in my freezer, I can almost guarantee that it will be empty and in the garbage by daybreak. And if by some miracle it survives the night, the mere knowledge that it's in there frozen and delicious will wreak havoc on my emotions. My sister, Debbie, has a vice in the form of Cheerios Breakfast Bars. She says that on any given night they will call out to her 200–300 times. That is, until she stopped keeping them in the house. Recovering alcoholics don't hang out in bars, so somebody trying to lose or maintain their weight shouldn't have ice cream, potato chips, or Cheerios breakfast bars lying around. It is at night, not morning, that our demons come out and fight for comfort food. Instead, feed that demon fruit (note: citrus fruits can keep you awake, but apples and pears would work better at this time of day). I understand that if you have children at home it may be even more difficult, but the less crap you keep in the house, the better off you will be.

## DON'T PACK YOUR BOWLING BALL

When you go to the beach, you don't pack your bowling ball, and when you go skiing, you don't bring your tennis racquet. The reason for this is simple: you don't need it. The same thought process should be applied each time you sit down for a meal. Think about what you'll be doing for the next two to three hours and then eat accordingly. If you'll be sitting at a desk and staring at a screen, you don't need a high-carb lunch. In that case, the majority of the nutrients should be protein and fat. But if you plan on lifting weights or going for a run, then load up on carbs and fuel a strong workout.

Being mindful of the short term allows you to make logical food choices that will keep your body operating at a high level. The timing of nutrients is crucial and will largely determine whether you will be fit or fat and full of energy or lethargy. Remember, eat for what are you are doing, not for what you have done.

## COOKING IS KING

Cooking is unlike singing because everybody can do it. While only 40 percent of the population can carry a tune, every one of us has the capacity to buy groceries, turn on an oven, and follow a recipe. Instead, we go out or go online and pay someone else to do it. The same laziness that keeps people from exercising also keeps them from cooking. Today, the average American spends only 27 minutes a day on food preparation but sits for for five hours in front of a television, often watching someone else cook. Less than 60 percent of meals eaten at home were actually cooked there, while thirty years ago, the number was closer to 75 percent.[3]

As cooking at home has decreased, the average American's weight has shot up. According to the Center for Disease Control and Prevention, the average American woman today weighs 166 pounds, almost exactly the same as the average man weighed in the early 1960s.[4] Men have let themselves go even more, weighing nearly 30 pounds more today than they did in the 1960s. In a 2003 study, Harvard economist David Cutler found that when we do not have to prepare meals, we eat more of them. As the time cooking has decreased by half, we have added half a meal to our diet.[5]

When you don't prepare your food, you have no idea what you are eating. Even if the food appears healthy, the fish could be fried, the broccoli buttered, and the potato covered in salt. It is time to rise up off of the couch and cook once again like we did when *Leave It to Beaver* was on TV.

Here are some of the benefits of cooking at home:

- You will save a lot of money. Buying in bulk helps, too, so you have the ingredients for more than one meal!
- You will lose weight. When you control the ingredients, you control your body.
- Cooking at home encourages families to sit down and eat together and strengthens the bond between family members.
- You will appreciate and savor the food more, since you prepared it.
- You control portion size, which is usually far too large at restaurants.
- Your love life will thrive. Few things are a bigger turn-on than a nice person who can cook.

## WRITE IT DOWN

When I lift weights, I often see guys at the gym complete a set of an exercise and then pick up a pen and notebook and start writing. I imagine that they are logging the weights and reps of each exercise, but for all I know, they could be scribbling affirmations such as "I'm ripped!", "I'm huge!", and "I'm the sexiest man alive." If I am correct in my assertion, I applaud their behavior but recommend that they do this after the workout. Regardless of what they are recording, the constant start and stop disrupts the flow of the workout and makes them take longer rest periods than they necessarily need. Our brains are powerful enough to store those numbers for an hour before relaying them into a marble notebook. However, the same cannot be said for a food journal. These should be updated throughout the day when you are trying to lose weight. The reason for this is simple: calories are easily forgotten as the day goes on. That handful of nuts that you grabbed on the way out of the house does not exist unless you write it down. Tracking your diet has never been easier with the advent of great diet apps such as MyFitnessPal, My Diet Coach, and Calorie Counter—all available to download for free on your iPhone. Just enter the food you just ate, and the app will do the rest. I cannot tell you how many times a client has complained to me that he or she can't lose weight even though his or her diet has been squeaky clean. "I had a Greek yogurt for breakfast, salad for lunch, and some steamed vegetables for dinner." Yet somehow, the person gains two pounds! If you try to recall and write down everything you ate and drank at the end of the day, you're bound to forget something. You can lie to your trainer and nutritionist, but you can't lie to your digestive system. It remembers the steamed broccoli at dinner as well as the midnight bowl of Häagen-Dazs.

## CHEAT DAY

Once a week, I advise channeling your "inner Kobayashi" and eat like you'll never see food again. That's right, if it isn't nailed down, stick it in your mouth and chew. I'm talking pizza, ice cream, potato chips, cookies, spoonfuls of peanut butter, plates of pasta, and loaves of bread. Throw in a few margaritas and ten or fifteen beers and then pass out on the couch.

This is your "cheat day," and you will enjoy all of your cravings from the past six days of healthy eating. And if you can fit it all into one meal, even better. The point is to satisfy the craving and then return to your normal diet. When your body is conditioned to eating only healthy food, any meal high in saturated fat or sugar will make you feel like garbage shortly after eating it. This is why I recommend splurging on the weekend so you wake up slowly the next morning from your food coma. Now, if you don't have cravings, hold off on the meal until you do. And whether that's a week or a day away, when the craving comes, give into it.

---

**TAKEAWAYS**

- Plan a cheat day each week to avoid feelings of guilt and shame when you choose to eat something delicious.
- If you fall off track with your diet, focus on the next meal and get back on course.
- When you sit down to eat, think about what you'll be doing for the next two to three hours. If you'll be physically active, have a high-carb meal, but if you'll be stuck behind a desk, eat mainly protein and fat.
- Eat your biggest meals at breakfast and lunch and have a light dinner.
- The earlier you eat dinner, the better. Try to eat dinner at least three hours before bed to maximize sleep and digestion.
- Don't keep ice cream in the freezer or chips and candy in the pantry. Don't bring it home.
- Cook in bulk as often as possible with healthy food that will last you several days.

---

# CHAPTER 3
# Thomas Jefferson Was Wrong

## FAT SHAMING

Ever since I was a kid, I loved to eat. By third grade, I outweighed my fellow classmates by fifty pounds, and to be clear, it was not muscle that filled my prepubescent frame. Late at night, I'd chow down on bagels with cream cheese and endless bowls of cereal almost always washed down with several glasses of Mott's Apple Juice. As delicious as it sounds, that was my secret formula for weight gain: stuff myself with sugar and then go right to bed. Little did I know that I was ahead of my time, as millions of Americans now follow this eating plan, which explains the obesity epidemic in this country. When we had pizza once a week, it was

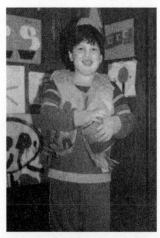

*Ready for the Thanksgiving feast.*

not unusual for me to eat four slices. Several times in my life, I devoured the entire pie, with plenty of room left over for dessert. My insatiable appetite and rotund stature caused me emotional and physical pain, as my parents and classmates "fat-shamed" me long before the title was fashionable. My parents were thin, fit health fanatics and never let me forget that I wasn't. Tired of being a 12-year-old punching bag with the outline of a garbage can, I joined the local gym and even lied on the membership application, claiming that I was 13, the minimum age to work out. Since I had very few friends, the gym became my sanctuary, and every day after school, I would head over to attack the weights. It was a healthy, aggressive activity that I could do alone and had complete control over. Rather than sit in my bedroom with the door closed playing video games, I surrounded myself with weights, mirrors, and other gym members. Some of the powerlifters there took me under their wing and gave me advice on how to build up my strength. When I was Bar Mitzvahed a year later, I was no longer obese and even had a semblance of muscle tone. I bought and read every muscle magazine and bodybuilding book that I could find and learned quickly about the importance of training and nutrition. Four years later, I had gone from being called "Fat Boy" and "Porker" as a kid to "Muscles" and "Meat" by my classmates in college. Still objectified, at least now I was beef instead of pork.

The simple act of lifting weights supplied me with a new-found sense of confidence, taught me the benefits of hard work, and gave me a healthy, muscular physique.


## VANITY

Vanity is the number-one driving force that brings people to the gym to lift weights and run on a treadmill. Sure, if exercise helps them live a longer, healthier life, that's also nice, but nobody has ever received a compliment on a first date for their slow pulse or low blood pressure. "Oh my God, your cholesterol is amazing" is something that you will never, ever hear. But "Michelle Obama arms" and "six-pack abs" have been cemented into our vernacular by mainstream media. Even workout clothes are now designed to bring out the very best a physique has to offer. Look at any woman's butt in Lululemon yoga pants and the same butt in Nike yoga pants, and it tells two very different stories. Men are just as deceptive! Instead of that old, stained t-shirt from college, men now work out in 100-dollar micro-fiber, high performance gear t-shirts designed to enhance their low-performance, couch-potato physique. Rather than rely on fancy fabric and deceptive design, why not create a physique that looks incredible both in and out of clothes?

In a world where there so are few things that we have control over, it's a shame to let your body go to waste. What you eat and drink, the frequency and intensity of your exercise, and how much sleep you get will largely determine how you look and feel. To control one's body means having the ability to sculpt the silhouette that will follow you everywhere. Sure, we all have genetic limitations, but why not test the physical waters and see what our bodies are really capable of? We'll spend thousands of dollars on clothes and tens of thousands on a fancy car to enhance our appearance, but not forty-five minutes a day in a gym? Yes, Andrew, that is correct. Cars and clothes can be purchased in under a minute with a credit card, while a great physique takes hard work, discipline, and years to develop. Though vanity brings people to the gym, the psychological benefits are anything but shallow. These include greater self-esteem, less stress, and a lower risk of Alzheimer's Disease and many types of cancer.

## THOMAS JEFFERSON WAS WRONG

Despite what Thomas Jefferson said, all men are not created equal. We're not! We're tall, short, smart, stupid, skinny, fat, bald, hairy, scrawny, stocky, and muscular. We have genetic limitations and must accept and work with them. After all, what choice do we have? Actually, today we can just go to the plastic surgeon and place an order: "Yeah, Doc, give me a bigger chest, a flat stomach, a round ass, and diamond-shaped calves, please. And if there's any money left over, go ahead and fix my nose and remove that mole that I thought was a birth mark." Or you can do it the natural, inexpensive way and go to the gym. Given the worst genes for muscle growth, I have been able to add 90 pounds of muscle to my frame. I'll never have giant calves or a gorilla chest, but I'll be the leanest guy in the gym. Never a mass monster, I train for symmetry and proportion.

Your genetics are not your fault, but they are your responsibility. When you look into the mirror, take stock of what you see and paint the best picture in your mind that you can. Then go to gym and work toward creating that body. If you're born with narrow shoulders, you may choose to work on widening your back, streamlining your waist, and developing your outer quad sweep. If you're born with wide hips, you may want to work on your glutes, hamstrings, and side delts. If you are born with tiny calf muscles, perhaps your goal is to blast them into oblivion until they grow. Shaping your unique frame with specific exercises is no different from wearing braces to improve your smile. Most important, do not compare yourself to other people because unlike cars, no two bodies are identical. In the wise words of Theodore Roosevelt, "Comparison is the thief of joy."

## PICK YOUR POISON

In the 1940s, American psychologist William Sheldon took measurements of naked Ivy League students and declared three different body types—ectomorphs, mesomorphs, and endomorphs.

Here's the rundown:

**Ectomorph**: The pencil-neck geek who gets the shit kicked out of him in school (i.e., Peter Parker, me). We have to fight for every ounce of muscle. Genetics say "skinny." We say "strong"!

**Mesomorph**: The high school quarterback. He's built like a brick shithouse and gets all the girls, as well as their sisters. He merely has to look at a weight, and muscles magically appear.

**Endomorph:** The fat guy who holds the money during a bet. Both of his parents are large mammals (soft, round, with thick bones). Genetics say, "fat." He says, "feed me."

Identify your own body type and then tailor your training around it. Many of you are likely a combination of two of these body types, all of which have their benefits and limitations. The endomorph has to do hours of cardio to lose weight, while the ectomorph just has to stare at a treadmill, and unwanted weight melts away into thin air. The mesomorph comes within ten feet of a bench press and his pecs pump up, while the ectomorph has to train like a madman to gain a quarter inch on his chest. You can thank your parents for whatever hurdles you have to overcome, but luckily, there is always a way to improve. Studies have shown that most of us burn within 300 calories of one another, so metabolically, we are not as different as we appear.[1] You may have to work twice as hard and eat half as much as your skinny friend, but don't use that as an excuse to sit at home and do nothing. Put in the work and you will be rewarded. That much I can guarantee.

## THE HIGH-FASHION DIET

There has long been a myth that a supermodel's diet consists solely of cocaine and cigarettes. In recent years, scientists have added Diet Coke to that equation. In reality, most models meet the body mass index for anorexia. Twenty years ago, the average model weighed 8 percent less than the average woman.[2] Now, they weigh 23 percent less, and the number is rising faster than China's population. Plus-size models used to range from sizes 12 to 18. Now, they're between sizes 6 and 14. The average runway model is 5'11", 114 pounds, with no boobs, butt, or body fat. The clothes are meant to dangle on their body like a hanger, as the human mannequin struts down the catwalk with a blank stare and a growling breadbasket. If you weren't anorexic before watching a runway show, you will be afterwards. These emaciated women are literally dying to be thin. "Anorexia may be the most talked about illness among models, but bulimia is probably the more common," says Dr. Adrienne Key.[3] "Size zero" became front-page news in September 2006, when model Luisel Ramos collapsed on a runway during Uruguay's Fashion Week and later died from heart failure that some thought to be related to anorexia. The list of models who have succumbed to anorexia is a long one.

With their long legs, wide-set eyes, and high cheekbones, these models influence girls as young as six years old to strive to resemble them. Each year, a new reality show airs where extremely average-looking women chase their dream of being a high-fashion model. This dream quickly dissipates and becomes a nightmare when they're told that they need to lose 10 pounds or that they are just not photogenic. Why open yourself up to such shallow subjectivity? Free yourself from that "anorexic cyclone" that sucks you in and spits you out. Finally, as a straight male, I think I speak for most men when I say that the "runway model body" is unattractive. Ladies, kill your inner supermodel! Kill her! Grab a baseball bat and bash her like a piñata. You're perfect, she isn't. Real women have curves—big, beautiful curves that say, "Hey baby, want to dance?"

## CURVES ARE SEXY

In a recent study, *Glamour Magazine* surveyed over 300 women of all shapes and sizes and found that 97 percent of them admitted to having an "I hate my body" moment every single day.[4] There are numerous explanations for this high number of women with a negative body image. Here are a just few of them:

1. Her parents fucked her up. My dad used to call me "fat boy." I'd be naive to think women get any less.
2. Her dickhead boyfriend told her to lose a few pounds even though she looks like a model.
3. She reads *Cosmo* and *Vogue*, where the models are 6 feet tall and weigh 100 pounds. Rule: if you can wrap your fingers around her thigh, she's too thin.
4. Her girlfriends tell her that she looks "healthy."
5. She watches *The Real Housewives*, in which the women constantly criticize their own bodies and get "work" done to fix imperfections.
6. She just ate pizza and ice cream.
7. She has a "fat" mirror and fluorescent lighting.

8. She shrunk her clothes in the dryer.

9. She's on her period.

10. She's pregnant.

## WEIGHT LOSS ON TV

When did one's ability—or lack thereof—to lose weight become exciting enough to put on television? As I continue to ask this question, shows like *The Biggest Loser* continue to expose overweight men and women who are being overworked. While the world watches, the competitors are seen panting, and sometimes even in tears. As a personal trainer, I firmly believe that there is no crying in weight loss. Lose it or don't lose it, but don't cry about it. It should never be that painful.

Like a prize fighter at Caesar's Palace, each contestant on *The Biggest Loser* steps on a scale in front of a mass audience, and the winner is the one who loses the highest percentage of bodyweight. Now in its 17th season, the show has continued to grow in popularity, and remarkably, U.S. obesity rates have also soared in the past 17 years, leaving 37 percent of the population obese.[5]

We see the weight loss on the TV show, but not the weight gain when the cameras are shut off, trainers are gone, and the competition is no longer against other people, but with themselves. In a recent *New York Times* article, scientist Kevin

### Weight Loss Reality Shows on TV
### (2004–present)

| | | |
|---|---|---|
| The Biggest Loser | Extreme Weight Loss | I Used to be Fat |
| Thintervention | Fit to Fat to Fit | Dance Your Ass Off |
| Heavy | Fat Chance | Weight Loss for Love |
| Celebrity Fit Club | Ruby | Operation Osmin |
| My Diet is Better Than Yours | Shedding for the Wedding | Money Hungry |

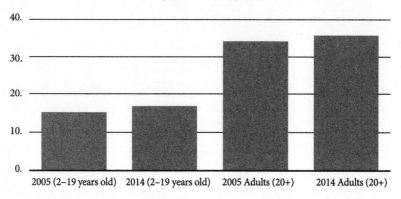

Obesity Rates in 2005 and 2014
(Source: CDC)

Hall tracks 14 *Biggest Loser* contestants for six years after their appearance on the show. The results of the study showed that 13 out of the 14 contestants had gained back most of their weight.[6]

The growing number of weight-loss shows on television is a direct result of the food and beer commercials shown during the break. Television may not necessarily be the cause of obesity, but it's definitely an ally. When was the last time you saw a commercial for carrots or bananas? The second this country removes processed food from their diet and treats exercise as a lifestyle—not as a crash course—there will be no more obesity and no need for these shows.

## MANOREXIA

Eating disorders plague seven million women and one million men in this country.[7] Today, men are subjected to male mannequins with 27-inch waists.[8] Fifty years ago, the same company's mannequins had 33-inch waists. Will somebody put some wood on these fuckers?

In many cases, a grown man with a 27-inch waist is suffering from manorexia. Men's magazines always showcase the guy with the perfect body on the cover, and some men feel social pressure to look like that. Some want to be wiry like Steven Tyler, ripped like Brad Pitt, or massive and cut like *People* Magazine's 2016 Sexiest Man Alive, Dwayne "The Rock" Johnson. To get those six-pack abs, they figure, "Screw it, I just won't eat." What they hoped would give them a washboard stomach actually makes it protrude due to low-plasma levels, which cause a leakage of fluid out of the blood vessels and into the stomach.

Several male celebrities—including Dennis Quaid, who sought treatment for his disorder after losing 40 pounds for a movie—have come forward to admit that they suffer from manorexia. Billy Bob Thornton also lost 59 pounds in his own battle with the disorder.[9] The "King of Pop," Michael Jackson, was a mere 112 pounds when he died.[10] Standing 5'9", that would give him a BMI of 15.6. According to the World Health Organization, a BMI of 16.0 is the weight at which one might die of starvation.

Like women, men need to kill their inner "fitness model." Moderation is the key to living a healthy lifestyle. If your current diet and workout routine are not something that you can realistically sustain up until the day you die, then you're not doing it right. A zero-carb diet is just as bad as a hardcore powerlifting workout that tests your one-rep max each day. Whether it is today, tomorrow, or two years from now, eventually you will get injured and become sick. Start today and eat and work out in a fashion that seems possible thirty years from now. That probably means no more 700-pound squats or 20-mile jogs through the park. That likely also means no more zero-carb diets or eating red meat every night for dinner.

In the extreme sport of professional bodybuilding, body dysmorphic disorder or "bigorexia" is rampant, and no matter how gargantuan competitors appear to the world, they are never big enough for themselves. This preoccupation with size and mass is the reason that anabolic steroids and growth hormones are so prevalent. Scores of bodybuilders have died in their thirties, forties, and fifties from long-term abuse of performance-enhancing drugs that prove toxic to the heart, liver, and kidneys. While competitive bodybuilding used to be an art form, it is currently a freak show where, in some cases, judges actually award the man who took the most drugs. The prize money and title only reinforce the abuse (e.g., the Mr. Olympia winner gets $250,000), and the champion might then take even more drugs to come back bigger the following year. Sadly, once they finish competing on stage, the body takes a sharp 180, and the health problems pile up quickly. Like with any other addiction, the bodybuilders need to stop obsessing over being the biggest he/she can be and should instead settle for a healthier, less massive physique that is still above average. Also, the skinny, vulnerable teenager who stares at these muscle freaks in magazines and dreams of attaining their look must be taught that it is unrealistic and extremely unhealthy. Muscle should only be gained naturally and gradually.

As a bodybuilder, I battle with my own body dysmorphia daily. I have also learned that nobody actually cares how muscular I am. To me, it is critical, but to my friends, it's frivolous. Being a good person is what really matters. Sadly, when your self-worth is dependent on maintaining a strong physique, depression intervenes when you suffer a setback. An injury occurs, you can't train for a few weeks, and you lose ten pounds of muscle and a big chunk of self-esteem. The bodybuilder mentality is a selfish affliction that pushes you away from balance when you focus too much on yourself. The intense training, strict diet, and focus inward can quickly cause you to withdraw from society and live only for your muscles. Only when you put other people first and your physique second do you stand a fighting chance at balance.

## STEROIDS

If I had a dollar for every time somebody offered me steroids, I could buy so much juice! Instead, I've spent that money on chicken breasts, protein powder, and gym memberships. The main reason that I have stayed drug-free for my 25 years in the iron game is that I never wanted to sacrifice my health for bigger muscles. Steroids are dangerous and illegal, and they shrink your testicles. Did you hear that last part? I mean, what else would you buy with that knowledge going in? If you found out a Honda Accord shrunk your testicles, you wouldn't buy one. No, you would buy the Volvo because it's safe. Some may not believe in judging other people's decisions to use performance-enhancing drugs, and I am not one of them. Unless you are a burn victim or fighting a disease that warrants the use of steroids, I am vehemently against them.

The tell-tale signs of steroid use are vast. They include puffy shoulders and traps, hair loss, acne, increased vascularity (skin-popping veins), and an overly aggressive personality. Far worse is what you don't see internally, as your organs work infinitely harder to process the synthetic testosterone that your body had no interest in producing on its own. In addition, most of those over the age of 45 who claim they have "Low T," in order to receive testosterone therapy, are simply ridiculous! They don't have low T, they're just 45! Their skin wrinkles, hair turns gray, balls sag, testosterone lowers, and metabolism slows down. Still, a 2013 study in the *Journal of the American Medical Assoiciation* found testosterone prescriptions have tripled since 2001.[11] Men over 45 take testosterone with the hope of looking and feeling younger and in doing so expose their otherwise healthy bodies to serious side effects. A *JAMA* study found that men who use testosterone therapy raise their chances of stroke, heart disease, and death by 30 percent.[11]

Over the years, I have been disheartened to learn that some of my childhood idols, such as Arnold Schwarzenegger and Hulk Hogan, were steroid users. When you are young and naive, you believe that the Herculean physiques you see on TV are built naturally. After all, Hulk Hogan did stare me down on television and say, "To all my little Hulkamaniacs, say your prayers and take your vitamins!" I now know exactly what he meant.

Then there is Lyle Alzado, a two-time Pro Bowl selection and linebacker on the 1984 Super Bowl Champion Los Angeles Raiders. Lyle Alzado, who graduated from Lawrence High School in the same class as my mother, died of brain cancer in 1992 at the age of 43. He attributed his illness to steroid abuse and spent the last years of his life advising teenagers to not make the same mistake he did. Here is an excerpt taken from a Lyle Alzado interview published in *Sports Illustrated*:

"I started taking anabolic steroids in 1969 and never stopped. It was addicting, mentally addicting. Now I'm sick, and I'm scared . . . all the time I was taking steroids, I knew they were making me play better. I became very violent on the field and off it. I did things only crazy people do." Alzado goes on to tell a story about a man who once sideswiped his car whom he, in turn, beat up. After describing his memory issues and hair loss, he subsequently states his last wish for no one else to die in the same manner as he did.[12]

## THE NATURAL PATH TO HEALTH

One mammoth truth that allows me to write so confidently about my training and nutrition is that unlike 99 percent of champion bodybuilders who have written books and published articles, I have never used steroids. Often lacking from these publications, but certainly necessary, is the inclusion of bodybuilders' diet and steroid cycles. This is because a chemically enhanced body drastically differs from a natural one and recovers much faster from workouts with much greater strength and endurance. If you doubt this fact, just compare the bodybuilding champions of today versus the Mr. America in 1955. You will perceive what appears to be two different species. The former is gargantuan with freaky size and vascularity, while the latter is eighty pounds lighter and much more aesthetic. One is pumped full of steroids, growth hormones, and plasma expanders, while the other was built on fish, fruits, and vegetables.

First and foremost, bodybuilding should improve your health, not destroy it. Remember, it's "bodybuilding," not "body-killing." Performance-enhancing drugs have taken this sport into a very ugly, dangerous direction, which is evident by all of the dead bodybuilders in recent years. Whereas Jack LaLanne won the 1955 Mr. America and lived an active life until the ripe old age of 96, modern bodybuilders today suffer heart attacks in their forties and fifties and rarely make it to sixty. More impressive than 20-inch arms matched with 4 percent body fat is the healthy medley of happiness and longevity.

## HOW TO MEASURE PROGRESS—THE SCALE

A scale is like a narcissistic parent that consistently makes you feel bad, so please, limit contact to a maximum of once a week. If you step on a scale each morning, you provide it the power to wreak havoc on your emotions and make your mood swing back and forth like a pendulum. If you lose two pounds, you will feel like the stars are aligned and walk with your head held high. But gain back three, and you'll want to stick that same head in the oven. Worse is that the number tells you nothing about body composition! It provides no information about important details regarding muscle, fat, bone composition, or water content. While a digital scale may accurately determine weight, its attempt to measure body fat is completely inaccurate. If you step on a digital scale three times in one day, there's a good chance your body fat percentage will fluctuate 10 to 20 percent. Factors such as how hydrated you are and the last time you ate and exercised all play a role in the faulty body fat reading. At 7 a.m., you may be 22 percent body fat, at 9 a.m., 29 percent, and amazingly at 10 p.m., you're a whopping 44 percent! You stand there in your underwear staring at that number thinking, *Should I kill myself now or later?* If you cannot emotionally handle stepping on a scale, use the mirror as your guide, take lots of photos, and observe the way your clothes fit. They will tell you everything you need to know.

## BODY FAT TESTING

The number that discloses the most information about your fitness level is body fat percentage. Unfortunately, the methods to gauge this number are not always reliable. The most popular and convenient technique used is the skin-fold test. When I worked at Equinox in 2002, I had to pinch prospective clients with the skin fold caliper and can honestly say that the numbers I presented were far from reliable. I would grab fat from different areas of their body with calipers that I could barely operate and then come up with a number that was optimistic yet conceivable. In hindsight, had I been a smart businessman, I realize that I should have taken that number and added 5-10 percentage points in order to fat-shame the client into believing that they needed a trainer. "I'm 43 percent body fat! My God, let's do five sessions a week until I get this under control." For an accurate measure of body fat, a DEXA scan is an x-ray that not only tells you body fat percentage, but also breaks down where it is stored in the body. Some universities with exercise physiology research programs will offer them to the public. Otherwise, you have to go to a radiologist or private lab, which usually costs $60 to $100. Then there is hydrostatic weighing, in which you stand on a scale in a swimming pool and compare that number to your normal weight plus the density of water. In other words, unless you have a nearby lab with a swimming pool at your disposal or go with the DEXA scan, forget body fat testing altogether.

## MIRROR, MIRROR

Better than a scale, body mass index, or body fat test is the good old mirror. The beauty of the mirror is that it does not provide you with a number, but an image. When a gym member sees a guy with freaky muscle development and vascularity checking himself out in the mirror and posing, he or she assumes that this is a classic case of narcissism and self-worship. While 99.9 percent of the time they are correct, the remaining .1 percent portrays a physique artist scrutinizing his work and using the mirror as his editor. It is no different from the woman who struts down the sidewalk and checks herself out in the reflection of the glass display window of a clothing store. Bodybuilders also take photos every couple of weeks to monitor their progress. Between mirrors and photos, you will see exactly what needs work and, more important, the progress that you have made. In the case of muscle development, an image provides you with much more information than a lump sum. And if you are dead set on numbers, a tape measure will tell you more than a scale.

---

**TAKEAWAYS**

- Kill your inner supermodel. Never compare yourself with others or let your body define you.
- If you are dating or married to someone who constantly criticizes your body, ask them to stop. If they continue, throw their clothes out the window and dump them.
- No matter how bad your genetics are, there is always light at the end of the tunnel. Put in the work in the kitchen and at the gym, and you will be rewarded.
- Never take any performance-enhancing drugs to develop your physique. They will kill you. Build muscle naturally and gradually.
- Use the mirror as your guide and take pictures. The scale tells you very little about body composition, while images show you everything.

# CHAPTER 4
# Gym Fashion and Etiquette

When I work out, I wear a solid-colored t-shirt and warm-up pants—plain, boring, and comfortable. While I don't go to the gym to compare my wardrobe with that of the other members, I can't help but notice how awful people can look given the wrong dress. Let's explore a few of these fashion woes:

**Men**
**Jogging shorts** – Unless you're a Kenyan or a kickboxer in Thailand, you shouldn't be wearing these.

**Wife beaters** – You look like pure trash.

**Sleeveless self-cut t-shirt** – There's a reason that t-shirt had sleeves, so don't make an art project out of it. Buy a sleeveless shirt if that's your style.

**Shin-high tube socks** – Nothing makes you look like an old Jewish man more than knee-high tube socks pulled down halfway by the shin. Go with low-cut socks or wear pants over your knee-highs.

**Stringy muscle tank** – This hasn't been in style since the late '80s. Still, some men actually wear these things and look ridiculous.

**White undershirts with dirty armpits and stains** – You look like a homeless person.

**Construction boots** – You're not hunting, Buzz. Buy some Nikes.

**Vibram Lizard Sneakers** – Shaped to match your feet, the neon Vibram "FiveFingers" make you look like an asshole and an amphibian all at the same time.

**Flip-flops** – Straight from the beach to the gym, this guy is one dropped dumbbell away from learning a very important lesson.

**Sunglasses** – Like Larry David said, "You know who wears sunglasses inside? Blind people and assholes."

**Jeans** – It's not a bar, moron. Get an elastic waist like a normal human being.

## Women
**Oversize team-building t-shirts with holes** – The old J.P. Morgan Challenge t-shirt that she got in 2004 is still three sizes too big and has mustard stains all over it.

**Pants that promote camel toe** – One pair of lips in the gym will do just fine.

**Cutoff shirts** – Unless you have a tight stomach and lower back, this look can be disastrous.

**Sports bras, without a shirt over them** – Again, your stomach and lower back better be tight, or this won't work. Remember, you don't want to be that person in the gym about whom other people whisper, "Wow, she's so brave to wear that."

**Saggy pants** – Nobody likes a saggy ass. Wear something that hugs your butt.

**In full makeup** – It's a gym, not a wine bar.

Note: As much as I loathe the idea of $100 yoga pants and what they represent, such clothes look good. Brands like Lululemon have figured out a way to make every woman's ass look tighter and boobs look bigger. In other words, their stuff is gold.

When you dress for the gym, please take these ideas into account. Aim to blend in or stand out in a good way. Don't become famous for your camel toe.

## GYM ETIQUETTE

The following people should have their gym memberships revoked:

**The Stinker** – The guy who wears dirty gym clothes and no deodorant, and smells like a rotting dog, He ends up with half the gym to himself, as nobody can go within 40 feet of his rancid stench.

**The Grunter** – The meatheaded shitstack who didn't get enough love as a kid and sounds like he's giving birth. I want to throw a 45-pound plate in this guy's mouth.

**The Dumbbell Clanker** – This idiot needs closure on each repetition, so he clanks the dumbbells together and produces a horrible, piercing, dog-whistle noise. I once asked this juiced-up meathead why he clanked the dumbbells together. He said, "To align the Universe." I said, "Carry on, then."

**The Supersetter** – The one who simultaneously uses the bench press, leg press, lat pulldown, and squat rack, putting a towel down on each so as to reserve each piece of equipment. Pick one, asshole.

**The Sweat Slob** – The one who perspires all over a bench and then walks away without wiping it up.

**The Hover Craft** – The pest who hovers around you and waits for you to finish up. You feel pressured, rush your set, and get nothing out of it. You just want to scream, "Get the fuck out of here!"

**The Water Hog** – The one who fills up his 10-gallon tank and keeps you salivating in need of a swig.

**The Socializer** – He knows everyone's name and comes up to you midset and says, "Haven't seen you in awhile." And you're thinking, "Yeah, it wasn't long enough." I mean, my head is down and my music is blasting because I clearly want to chat.

**The Don Juan Trainer** – The sleazy, dumb trainer that goes up to all the girls and says, "You're doing this wrong," in a tone that screams, "I want to fuck you." Don't hire him. Report him to management.

**The Man in Medical Scrubs** – Ladies, the doctor has arrived! Too busy to change out of his scrubs, Superman flew straight from the operating room to the bench press. In the process, he spread a new strain of E. coli on the equipment. Thanks, Doc.

**Mr. Ivy League** – The guy wears a Harvard t-shirt, Yale shorts, and Princeton hat to show off his large brain. Save your Ivy League flair for the reunion.

**The Battle Ropes Clown** – This person takes up 30 feet of gym space playing lasso with those thick ropes that swing up and down and to the side in different patterns for no reason. You could do all of the same movements with five- or 10-pound dumbbells in each hand and take up hardly any space.

**Phone Call on Treadmill** – Nobody wants to hear your conversation. Period. Thank God for headphones!

**The Guy Flexing in the Mirror** – Save this for your bathroom.

**The Guy who Used to Look Like That** – "I used to look like you!" Sure, you did.

**The Refuse-To-Rack-Weights Guy** – If you can pick it up, you can put it back.


## WHAT TO BRING TO THE GYM?

**Food** – If you're coming straight from work, pack an apple or banana to eat right before your workout. And if you're not going straight home after a workout, pack a protein shake with you.

**A water bottle** – Drinking water during a workout is a must, but don't be one of those clowns who walks around with a gallon of water in his hand like he's preparing for a flood.

**Headphones** – Whether it's Beatz by Dre or cheap earbuds that you bought for two bucks on a flight home from Cleveland, the ability to block out annoying gym noise is a must. The clanking of dumbbells, slamming together of 45-pound plates, primal grunting, and choleric roar of "All you, two more, you got this!" is enough to send you rummaging through your gym bag for aspirin. As for the actual music, gyms tend to play Top 40 hits, but I suggest you make your own playlists to score your workout as you see fit. Also, time the playlist so that it lasts you through your full workout. No repeating songs! Some old-school folks argue that music distracts you from the workout, and that is precisely why I believe music is a necessity. The more you think about doing your crunches, the more aware you are of your breathing, and the less likely you are to continue. In a 1999 study, music was shown to facilitate exercise performance by reducing the sensation of fatigue, increasing psychological arousal, promoting relaxation, and improving motor coordination.[1] So, whether you prefer country, rap, or classic rock, these jukebox heroes will add weight to your bench press and speed up your mile, and tighten up your body.

**Weight belt** – If you're planning on doing heavy deadlifts, squats, overhead presses, shrugs, standing curls, or lateral raises, definitely purchase and use a leather lifting belt to protect your lower back. However, don't use it as a crutch and make sure to take it off for exercises that don't call for the necessary support. Allow your core muscles to stretch and contract as often as possible.

## A GYM FOR ALL WALKS OF LIFE

People who claim that they hate the gym need to shop around more and generalize less. In gyms, atmosphere is everything, and thankfully, they cater to all walks of life. If you seek attention and enjoy a fashion show with high-end machines, eucalyptus-scented locker rooms, and plush towels, there is a gym for you. If you prefer less of a scene and choose to lay low and blend in with decent equipment and a friendly staff, there is also a gym for you. If you're an iron addict and crave a bare-bones, hard-core gym with rusty free weights, heavy metal music, and muscleheads shooting up in the bathroom stall, I suggest you wash your hands constantly, and, yes, there's a gym for you. If you're a woman and insist on only working out around other women, there's a gym for you. If you're extremely frugal and don't mind mismatched weights, dirty benches, and homeless people using the locker room to shower, fear not; there's a gym for you, too.

Unless you feel you're being brutally ripped off, don't sweat the price. A good gym is a great investment.

For the antisocial butterflies who do not enjoy sweating around other people, I suggest you go to the gym when it is the least crowded—from 5:30 to 7 a.m., 10 a.m. to noon, or 2 p.m. to 4 p.m. If you have an hour free within any of these windows, you'll have to interact less and get a better workout. Personally, a superpacked gym is my idea of hell. Not only does it mean having to wait for equipment, but it also involves interacting with the gym members who seem to want to do whatever you're doing at the same time. Even in a near-empty gym with only two or three other people present, you can rest assured that one of them will ask to "work in" with you on an exercise. In a gym, every neurosis is on display. The one who failed to get enough love as a kid is grunting to the heavens, while the hot blonde with low self-esteem stretches in booty shorts by the power rack. The paranoid schizophrenic walks and talks to himself on the treadmill, and the woman with severe OCD puts towels on every piece of equipment available.

If you enjoy a loud, overcrowded bar, then you belong at the gym at 6 p.m., when the after-work crowd arrives. An excellent pickup spot, the gym is a place at which many relationships develop and where endorphins are high and clothing is kept to a minimum. A simple "Are you using this?" is an easy way to strike up a conversation, followed by "I see you here all the time. I'm Doug, by the way. We should get a drink sometime." And then she says, "No thanks, I have a boyfriend," and you walk away with your tail between your legs.

## NO INITIATION FEE
When you join a gym, the salesperson will tell you that there is a onetime initiation that has to be paid with your membership.

This fee is typically equal to the cost of one or two months and is an absolute scam. Do not pay this fee! Gyms have no business charging an initiation fee, because there is nothing to initiate. They are not running cable wires through your wall or installing a satellite dish on your roof. It's a gym, and all of the equipment and amenities are already there. Tell them, "Thank you, but I'm not joining if I have to pay an initiation fee." Then they'll pretend to check with their supervisor, agree to your demand, and ten minutes later, you're doing dips to Guns N' Roses.

## THE REST PERIOD SELFIE

Before Smartphones, the gym was a place that people went to to work out, socialize, and stare at themselves in the mirror. Like brushing your teeth, exercise was a habit that was performed daily and kept to yourself. Staring at yourself in the mirror, which was considered shallow and self-indulgent then, now appears modest by comparison, in today's social media-driven universe, where meatheads in Under Armour upload selfies every five minutes with hashtags such as #shredded, #gainz, #gymrat, and #beastmode. Once upon a time, rest period meant a time to catch your breath in preparation for the next set. Now, it is an opportunity to interrupt another person's workout and ask them to take a picture of you flexing. Sometimes they'll even ask you to retake the photo because a few dozen "Likes" on Instagram depend on it. When I am approached and asked to play photographer, I respectfully decline. After all, why encourage this behavior? Make the idiot shoot into the mirror like any well trained, self-sufficient narcissist.

It is my belief that anyone who takes a "selfie" in the middle of their workout and posts it on social media should be thrown out of the gym and then defriended on Facebook. That includes takng screenshots of the mileage of your run, the video of your deadlift, and the spin class that you took at 6 a.m. with the hashtag "#roosters." Save the uploading for when you leave the gym or, better yet, keep it to yourself. Remember, your friends do not care about your workout.

## EAT TOGETHER, EXERCISE ALONE

On a beautiful Sunday morning in June, I walked through Central Park and noticed a couple in their early thirties running side by side in holy matrimony. The patriarch was shirtless, and his damsel was wearing a sports bra. They might as well have been holding hands, and I thought, *My God, take a break!* Soon enough, you can play footsie on the couch and watch "Big Brother" while you cross chopsticks and feed each other brown rice sushi. Though I may sound like a "Debbie Downer," I think it's important for a couple not to do every single activity together. When I was a kid, my parents played tennis against each other on the weekend, and it was always catastrophic. Since they were both talented players and super-competitive, whoever lost would accuse the other of cheating, and my dad, with the on-court temperament of John McEnroe, would throw his racquet in frustration. They would make a scene and then drive home together in silence or, far worse, curse each other out all the way back to the house. They kept this pattern of behavior up throughout my childhood and in doing so taught me a very valuable lesson: do not compete in activities against your spouse. Be their partner in doubles, but never their opponent in singles. If you go to the same gym, walk in together and then part ways once you pass the front desk.

Like competitive sports, working out together in the gym is a recipe for disaster. I have seen many couples try this, and it rarely lasts more than a few workouts before it comes to an abrupt end. First of all, the two lovebirds may have opposite goals. He may want to build muscle mass, while she wants to lose five pounds. Chances are that their strength levels are not even, which creates an internal strife and feelings of inferiority in the weaker of the two. Typically, the guy shows off how strong he is to his girlfriend, as she acts impressed and tactfully checks out the Greek god lifting twice as much weight two benches over. Her man further displays dominance when he corrects her form and starts bossing her around. This makes her feel even more insecure until she decides to never work out with him again and contemplates ending the relationship. A workout is an opportunity to focus on yourself and allow your mind and body to work in unison. For that hour, forget about everything else in your life, including your spouse. Eat together and exercise alone.

## FITBIT OR FREEDOM?

We began with calories, moved on to steps, and pretty soon, we will be counting our chews. Each time our teeth gnaw down on an apple and our jaw rotates, the "Chewbit" will log the motion and then vibrate once we have exceeded our 100-chew allotment. Of course, this device would be derivative of the popular "Fitbit" that monitors a person's steps and vibrates once you reach the 10,000-step goal. But what do 10,000 steps really tell you? Well, it tells you that you walked a cumulative distance of 5 miles. Did you do 4,000 of them in succession during a 30-minute walk? Or did you walk from the couch to the kitchen and back 1,000 times?

The stylish wriststrap is like a muted drill sergeant that constantly reminds you to get off your ass and move. As brilliant as this may sound, the *Journal of the American Medical Association* found that more than half of all Fitbit users throw it in a drawer after six months and never use it again.[1] Other consumers regifted the Fitbit to a friend or family member, who then regifted it to the neighbor next door.

Like a summer fling, a person and their FitBit are hot and heavy for a few months before the person seems to quickly lose interest. During the honeymoon phase, people become obsessed with their Fitbits and have friendly competitions with other people and their Fitbits. They become so infatuated with topping their personal best and beating their friends in "steps" that they start bragging to anyone that will listen. "I walked 20,000 steps today!" Go ahead and brag about your five-mile run if you must, but steps? That would be like a writer boasting about how many syllables he wrote. The Fitbit is similar to a deprivation diet due to the psychological impact it has on a person. "Mind your own business" is the consensus among users who abandoned the invasive device. The failure of the Fitbit to register other forms of exercise such as yoga and weight lifting also irritated consumers of the product. Rather than have a wristband run your life, take a walk, lift weights, or ride a bike for an hour. Once you are finished, eat a healthy meal and then wallow in freedom.

## IMAGINARY LAT SYNDROME

ILS, or Imaginary Lat Syndrome, became popular in the late 1980s when pro wrestling peaked and every guy wanted to be like Hulk Hogan. Instead of lifting weights and eating protein, they decided to walk like a bull, with their arms out to the side 20 to 40 degrees away from their body. This created an "I'm the man" type of feel in its earliest devotees and is still very popular in gym culture today. By holding your arms out to your side, you take up more space, but it does NOT make you look bigger. Any bodybuilder will tell you that by holding your arms out to the side like someone with ILS, you will destroy any lat width that exists. When striking a "Lat Spread" pose in competition, it's imperative to hold the hands tight into the waist. Now, if you don't have lats, that doesn't matter, and therein lies the value in ILS. More space means tougher—or so they think. I laugh when I see these deluded meatheads strut by me with their oversize egos. They finish their stellar approach with a face that yells, "What? You got a problem?" Women are constantly expose to ILS because it is known as the "pickup posture." Think of the film *Tommy Boy*, when Chris Farley says, "Do you know where the weight room is?" to the hot chick in the bikini. That's the walk I'm talking about! Men, please retire this march of bravado and walk like a normal human being.

# CHAPTER 5
# Cults of Fitness

Like Charles Manson, David Koresh, and Jim Jones, cult leaders populate the world of fitness, and whether they call themselves "Heaven's Gate," "Twelve Tribes," or "The Branch Davidians," the name must be catchy or the cult will not survive. Enter CrossFit, Soul Cycle, and Barry's Boot Camp, and you will find millions of Americans standing by their chosen sweatshop and worshipping their instructors as the messiah. Let's explore the most popular fitness cults.

**THE SOUL CYCLE EXPERIENCE**
There I sat on Bike #51 in the back corner of the room, farthest from the instructor and closest to the door. I was not there to burn 500 calories or add variety to my workout routine, but simply to satisfy my curiosity. For years, I have heard the hype and seen the women walking around in their Soul Cycle attire telling tales of triumph in spinning classes that promised to

flatten even the fittest warrior. With a name like "Soul Cycle," I was intrigued to see what metaphysical experience went on in the candlelit room behind the closed doors. With an open mind, I looked around the room and saw mainly women who were either stretching or peddling before the instructor began the class.

At 4:30 p.m. on the dot, Lindsay, the spinning instructor, stormed into the room like a bat out of hell and screamed at the top of her lungs into her microphone, "I don't know about you, but I'm here to get messy!" With that, the whole class erupted in exuberance, and it felt like a revolution was about to take place. She continued, "I want you all to open your heart and decide what you want to be in here today." At that moment, I took a deep breath, opened my heart, and decided that I wanted to be a guy on a bicycle. The music began blasting—a steady mix of Kanye, Eminem, and other artists belting loud, angry songs. After yelling instructions, she would add an exclamation point by screaming "Ow!" like Michael Jackson, nearly every ten seconds. It became old quickly, and my soul began to suffer. With basic movements such as standing and peddling, sitting and peddling, and doing triceps push-ups on the handle bar, I followed closely and listened to the woman in charge. About 20 minutes into the workout, we were told to grab the weights from underneath our seats and do kickbacks. When I found the weights, I was shocked to discover that they were one-pound dumbbells! After all, I've trained geriatrics with pulmonary disease and had yet to see a one-pound weight until today. As I struggled through the triceps exercise, I began losing faith in Lindsay and the Soul Cycle establishment. Every so often, she'd scream, "That's it, give it to me!" Then she would come around to each bike and look the person in the eye and yell, "Yeah!" Her intensity was too high for the activity of riding a bicycle, and she appeared to be someone who was either high on crystal meth or had downed six Red Bulls prior to class. As we did the various weight exercises while we peddled, Lindsay reminded us that "We do so much for other people, let's enjoy this privilege to do for ourselves."

The one constant instruction was "Turn your knob a quarter turn to the right," which controlled the bike's resistance. As my soul fought through this train wreck of a workout, I was shocked to hear the teacher abruptly say, "Namaste," which signified the end of the class. Firstly, isn't "Namaste" specific to yoga? Secondly, it felt as if we had just begun this 45-minute showdown, and now we were done? I asked the girl next to me, and she confirmed that we were, in fact, finished.

As I was leaving Soul Cycle, the front desk guy asked me if I enjoyed the class. I said, "No, not at all," and he was shocked and confused. I explained to him that I hardly felt like I had worked out and that the teacher screamed "Ow" far too many times. He offered me a free class with another instructor in another location and promised me that the class would be a great workout. Unfortunately, my soul had already been taken and would not be able to make it to the next class. Like so many other fads, the packaging appeared to far exceed the product, and customers drank it all up along with the Smart Water that was provided upon arrival.

After taking a class, I can confidently say that the appeal of Soul Cycle is not found in the mediocre, moderate-intensity, stationary bike workout, but in the atmosphere and social life that is provided. The room is dimly lit with "glamour lighting," the music is fast-paced, and the instructor screams words of encouragement that just ooze intensity. The women all know one another and wear Soul Cycle attire with the skull and crossbones logo and catchy slogans such as "Aspire to Inspire," "Athlete, Legend, Warrior," "Ride. Rinse. Repeat.," and my personal favorite, "Front Row," in reference to being front and center in the class. It's truly a scene, but then again, it's better than just sitting on the couch. If you enjoy riding a bike, save your soul and go to the park. You'll burn more calories, breathe fresh air, and nobody will scream at you unless you cut them off.

## CROSSFIT: THE NICKELBACK OF THE FITNESS WORLD

Is CrossFit dangerous, you ask? Consider this: Greg Glassman, the founder of CrossFit, recently bragged on *60 Minutes* that he has twelve lawyers on retainer. O.J. Simpson had eight during his trial. CrossFit is an orthopedic surgeon's wet dream because inexperienced lifters are thrown into a high-intensity workout with powerlifting movements without being taught the proper form or conditioned for that type of routine.

At the local CrossFit Box, I audited the Beginner WOD (Workout of the Day) class and witnessed thirteen participants (ten of whom were women) squatting with atrocious form and weights that were far too heavy. I introduced myself to the "Coach," who is in charge of all thirteen beginners, and he gave me a crash course on everything that I needed to know about the workout. Mind you, he gave me this spiel with his back to the class while they knocked out forced reps of squats with their spines bent forward, using every ounce of strength they could muster to lift their bodies up. This lack of focus on the coach's part told me far more than what actually came out of his mouth. In fact, even if he had laser-like focus on his disciples, it still would be impossible to correct the thirteen people squatting at once. As a personal trainer who works with one person at a time, the idea of monitoring thirteen people doing heavy squats, an exercise that requires the most intricate of form, is pure insanity. The WOD commanded the class to do squats for 6 sets of 3 reps. Yes, 3 rep sets since everyone in the class is training for the New York State Powerlifting Championships. When you cut down the reps to three, you rely more on the tendons than the muscles to do the work. As you may imagine, the risk of injury goes up exponentially as the weights get heavier and the reps get lower.

The next exercise was overhead squats, where the people held the bar fully extended over their head and then made their descent into a full squat. This, too, was done for super-low reps. I watched women and men struggle to stay upright and not fall backwards, thereby breaking their back. They continued this exercise for fifteen more minutes.

The "Coach" recommended that I do CrossFit three days a week to start out and then pointed to another area in the "Box" (what the CrossFit world calls its gym) where people were freestyling with barbells. He said, "On Sunday's, we have an "Open Gym," where people can come in and do whatever they want with the equipment." *Wow,* I thought. *That sounds almost like, well, every gym ever!* We moved on to pricing and it was $275 a month for unlimited workouts. By then, even if they had offered to pay *me* that money, I would not have come back. It was truly the most dangerous form of exercise that I have ever seen. Even strongmen who throw beer kegs over their head, lift atlas stones, and pull tractor-trailers are at a lower risk of injury than the CrossFitters doing triples on overhead squats.

Every morning, the founder of the biblical-sounding workout posts the WOD on his website for millions of disciples to follow. These workouts appear completely random, void of any logical program design, and though newbies are told to scale back their WODs (too much, too soon), CrossFitters take a sense of pride in completing the workout in its original form. The result can be torn tendons and ligaments and if by chance they don't injure themselves, they might leave behind a puddle of vomit that is strangely celebrated by some in the community, represented by an actual mascot with the name "Pukie the Clown." CrossFit prides itself on combining the different fitness disciplines to create the perfect workout. Unfortunately, mixing powerlifting movements like deadlifts with high rep sets of 40 is like mixing coffee and orange juice. According to Dr. Stuart McGill, a professor of spine biomechanics at the University of Waterloo, "the risk of injury from some CrossFit exercises outweighs their benefits when they are performed with poor form in timed workouts." He added "there are similar risks in other exercise programs. . . ."[1]

CrossFit is truly the "Nickelback of the fitness world." Like a vegan, it doesn't take long for someone who does CrossFit to tell you. One CrossFitter told me he was setting new PR's every day. I said, "PR's?" "Personal records." Ah, yes. CrossFit prides itself on raising a person's one-repetition max, which is fine if you are a 25-year-old athlete and have been weight training for ten years. But for a 45-year-old man with minimal experience to be maxing out on deadlifts each week is irresponible and idiotic. Just because he pulls 225 one day, doesn't mean he can try for 250, after a sleepless night in which his baby daughter keeps him up all night. Hopefully, he attempts and fails, and puts it down without injury. That is the best-case scenario.

After interviewing numerous CrossFitters, I can see why they enjoy it—almost like a religion, they are comforted with likeminded people on a quest for strength, fitness, and a new PR. They even have social events listed on a chalk board by the front entrance.

The cool Reebok sneakers and apparel that has the word "CrossFit" inscribed all over it, along with the colored plates, warehouse atmosphere, and powerlifting movements, all add a certain "badass" quality that the CrossFitters enjoy. Yet in twenty years, long after enough knees, hips, and shoulders have been shattered, expect CrossFit to be a lost memory in the world of fitness.

## THE ZUMBA MASSACRE

A physics exam in Chinese would have been easier than the Zumba class I tried. Like climbing a tree during a tsunami, it was over before it began. We started with a cool, fresh double sidestep with a clap, and I thought, *Awesome, this is my jam!* After twenty seconds of rocking the back-and-forth double sidestep, the teacher suddenly just freaked out! He did some "Walk Like An Egyptian" Bangles video move and then started spinning, shaking, and break-dancing all at once. It was like being in a Michael Jackson video without any knowledge of the song, beat, or choreography. I began laughing at how lost I was but made sure that I kept moving my feet. As they did more and more complicated moves, I laughed harder until I completely lost it when the instructor began twerking.

As I tried to follow the class, I quickly became a hazard to the room as I turned the wrong way and swung the wrong leg. After ten minutes of being lost deeper and deeper into the woods, I made a brash decision. For the rest of the class, every time I found myself out of step, I would return to the double sidestep clap until I was ready to try again. It worked. I felt better and better until I looked around and realized that all of the women and the token male across the room never missed a beat. They were all in cahoots and knew the drill. The instructor would signal to his leg and then change the move into some crazy "kick, spin, fly" thing that everyone did perfectly. They kept going more and more nuts with their bodies, and I kept doing my double sidestep clap.

Zumba was a 45-minute nervous breakdown that was humbling and humiliating, and I could not wait to leave the room. The instructor might as well have said, "Andrew, you don't get this move? You'll never get the next one, ha, ha, ha!"

## THE PHYSIQUE EXPERIENCE

Ever since I met my wife, she has sworn by a workout known as "Physique 57." Since her mind is logical and taste impeccable, I thought, "Why not, I'll check it out." At 1:45 p.m., I saw the 2 p.m. class was on the schedule at a local studio and bolted out of my apartment.

When I arrived out of breath at 2109 Broadway, I was pleased to find out that like "Single White Female," this showdown would take place in the scenic Ansonia building. I walked up to the 2nd floor, signed up for my workout, and the front desk girl said, "Don't be nervous. Take off your shoes, class is about to begin."

As I entered the studio, I realized that I was the only person in the class not wearing black socks. My dirty white tube socks made me instantly self-conscious, as did the fact that I was the only male in the room. It was seventeen women in Lululemon attire and a dude with dirty socks. The teacher welcomed me and then asked if it was my first time and bravely, I admitted that it was. She said, "Don't worry, you'll get through this," and told me to grab a pair of weights. Smart and sensibly, she suggested that I use the 10-pound dumbbells over the two-, five-, and seven-pound weights. Then it was game time! We started blasting shoulders with presses, biceps with hammer curls, and triceps with kickbacks. With the hammer curls, we were told to only go halfway down with the weight until she declared, "Five more, then you know what's coming? Full reps!" Those ten-pound, full-range hammer curls began to weigh on me, and just in time, she interrupted, "Down on the floor, pushups!" We did some pushups, both fast and slow, and our pecs were pumped!

Next was the Bar Method part of the workout where we grabbed a wooden beam, stretched out our spine, and then blasted our glutes and hips with some squat and lunge variations. My crappy tube socks kept slipping, and I felt like an idiot. We were told to take our volleyball and stick it in between our thighs and then to squeeze them. She said, "Squeeze those glutes!" Squeeze them!"

Then it was back on the ground for some serious hip thrusting and pelvic elongation. In a bridge, we thrust our pelvis up and down as hard as we could, with long strokes and short ones, until we all reached orgasm, and then were told to hold the pose for ten seconds with little pulses thrown in.

Before we got too comfortable, we were back on our feet for some sumo squats and some yoga-like lunge poses. Then she yelled, "Back on the floor!" and it was time to shred our abs, with lots of twisting crunches and some more pelvic thrusts that left us gasping for air. She told us, "Crunch with the beat of music," and my God, we did! Like a chorus line of Rockettes, we crunched in sync and absolutely killed it! All of our muscles had been dealt with, and we were ready to conquer the world. The teacher put on some "Hall and Oates," we did a few easy stretches, and then it was time to go home. I was sweaty, pumped, and my glutes were sore. Physique 57 is sex in socks with a wooden beam thrown in. It's kinky, tiring, and a lot of fun.

## BIKRAM YOGA

Why would anyone choose to exercise in 105 degrees like a slave in Egypt? I've asked myself that the handful of times that I've done Bikram Yoga. With its moist air, sweaty carpet, and rotten egg stench, the class should really be called "staph infection." The unremitting 90 minutes of torture that it takes to complete the same 26 postures can best be compared to a film that is 45 minutes too long in a movie theater in Thailand with no air conditioning. Devoted Bikram masochists explain their motivation as "If I can get through the feeling of Hell, I can do anything."

A recent *New York Times* article detailed the so-called benefits and claims of working out in intense heat and found that all benefits top out at 100 degrees. "Above that you're risking your health and safety," according to Douglas Casa, a kinesiology professor at the University of Connecticut. He also believes 86 degrees with 65 percent humidity is ideal for hitting the "sweat sweet spot."[2]

To be fair, my older sister, Debbie, is a Bikram Yoga instructor, and the practice has enhanced her life tenfold. She loves the heat, the students, and the serenity that she experiences during the Bikram Yoga practice, as well as the fitness benefits she enjoys afterwards. Her passion for Bikram Yoga is the same as mine is for pumping iron.

## FITNESS EVENTS

If social media has proven anything, it's that our appetite for attention is insatiable. As people walk the streets with their selfie sticks and iPhones, no scenery is too dull for what could potentially garner 50 "likes" on Instagram. Few things are done in private anymore, and that does not exclude exercise. We all have "friends" who are incapable of doing a workout without posting a picture or letting you know how many miles they just ran. The fact that you may not care is irrelevant, as it is the prospect of "posting" that fuels their workout. "Killed it in spin class!" "Killed it in CrossFit!" "Killed it at the gym!" You didn't kill anything. You exercised the way you are supposed to. Quit killing things.

Participating in a fitness event is a great way to draw attention to yourself on social media. Before Facebook and Instagram, there was only the marathon, triathlon, and Ironman, a long-distance triathlon. Now, there are over a dozen races and events to brag about that include the half marathon, 10K, 5K, Tough Mudder, Tough Mudder Half, Warrior Dash, Spartan Race, Spartan Beast, Rugged Maniac, Century Ride, CrossFit Games, and the Half-Ironman. These events bring in huge revenues, since each one requires an entrance fee, and in return the participant gets a medal, t-shirt, and 150 "likes" on Facebook. It is truly amazing how much faster people run when there is a number pinned to their chest.

While some of these races are harmless and fun, the extreme endurance events can put your health and even your life at risk. I believe that many of these races should be outlawed and that we'll look back in a hundred years and say, "Wow, that was really stupid. We lost a lot of good men and women."

## The Marathon

During the Greco-Persian War in 490 BC, a Greek messenger named Pheidippides ran 26.2 miles from the town of Marathon to Athens to relay the news of an Athenian victory in the Battle of Marathon and then abruptly dropped dead. Fast-forward 2,500 years, and now 55,000 people run the same distance that proved fatal for young Pheidippides annually on the first Sunday in November on the streets of New York City. So, in essence, shouldn't everyone die at the end of the race to pay proper tribute? Sadly, eight people do die each year running a marathon. The human body, and more specifically, the heart are not designed to run 26.2 miles in one shot. "If you go run for 20, 30, 40 minutes—that's fine. The body's kind of designed to do that," says Dr. Peter A. McCullough, MD, MPH, a cardiologist at the Baylor University Medical Center at Dallas. "But when you go run for four hours straight, the heart chambers of about a quarter of individuals can't tolerate it. The chambers start to dilate and the heart releases distress signals," he says.[2] "The likelihood of dying while running a marathon is about the same as having a fatal motorcycle accident," says Umesh Gidwani, MD, chief of Cardiac Critical Care at Mount Sinai Hospital in New York City.[3] For this reason, I don't ride motorcycles or run marathons.

Many may wonder why so many people voluntarily participate in such a masochistic race, especially since they are not competing to win. The answer is simple: to tell other people they did it. I say tell them anyway, nobody cares, nobody is checking, nobody gives a shit. Wow, you and 55,000 others ran 26 miles and didn't drop dead. Good for you. If they are not doing it for the attention, why pay an entry fee and wait until the first weekend in November to run the race? Wake up on a Tuesday in May, have a cup of coffee, a banana, a few glasses of water, and run 26.2 miles. Then go home, shower, and take a nap. Nobody needs to know. Every step of the marathon, people cheer and friends and family hold signs and wear t-shirts with the runner's name on it. "Go Brad! You can do it!" Once they reach the finish line, they are wrapped in tin foil like a baked potato, and a medal is placed around their neck that will remain there for at least two weeks. Throughout their 5-month-long training for the race, they provide daily updates and photos on social media and thank their friends who inspire them to go the distance. Once the race is over and the attention is gone, there is only one thing left to do: sign up for another one!

**The Half Marathon**

According to Running USA, the half marathon is the fastest-growing race in the country, which should not come as much of a surprise. Compared to the historic 26.2 mile version, the half marathon allows the runner to train half as hard, run half as far, and get all of the accolades. Personally, I think you should get half a medal, half a number, and half a t-shirt, but that probably would not go over well with at least half of the runners. But seriously, what else can you do halfway and still feel like a winner? If you pay half your rent, you don't get a medal, you get evicted. If you do half your SATs, you don't apply to Harvard, you apply to McDonald's. Wow, you ran a half marathon? I'll tell you what, I'm semi-impressed.

Still, a 13.1-mile run is far too long and can be dangerous for your heart. Studies have found that running for health is maximized with much less mileage. "It seems like the maximum benefits of running occur at quite low doses," said Dr. Carl J. Lavie, medical director of cardiac rehabilitation and prevention at the Ochsner Medical Center in New Orleans. "For most of us, running for 20 to 30 minutes, or about a mile-and-a-half to three miles, twice per week would appear to be perfect."[4]

## The Triathlon

Running is free, swimming is free, and riding a bicycle is free. But participating in a triathlon costs an average of $375 in the US. Add on travel expenses, hotels, training costs, and a high-quality bike, and you're looking at several thousand dollars. On the NYC Triathlon website, the event is listed as a 1500m swim, 40K bike, and 10K run. Unfortunately, here in America we do not use the metric system and have no idea what these distances mean. Always a public servant, I will provide the conversions that come out to approximately a 1-mile swim, 25-mile bike ride, and 6.2-mile run. Any one of those three legs is a full workout on its own.

The triathlon can also be extremely dangerous. For every 100,000 triathlon participants, there are 1.5 deaths, twice as many as with the marathon.[5] The majority of fatalities take place in the water during the first leg of the race. The competitor is full of adrenaline and panics from the hundreds of kicking feet and bodies swimming around him/her and goes into cardiac arrest. This is the complete opposite of the marathon, where the majority of deaths occur during the last mile, when the runner, full of adrenaline, sprints to the finish line and triggers an abnormal rhythm to an already susceptible heart.[6]

The risk involved in these endurance races needs to be considered before signing your life away. "People need to understand that they're not necessarily gaining more health by doing more exercise," said David Prior, a cardiologist and associate professor of medicine at the University of Melbourne. "The attributes to push through the barriers and push through the pain are common in competitive sport, but that's also dangerous when it comes to ignoring warning signs."[2]

Competing in a triathlon is a terrible way to die and has no Greek mythological significance like the marathon. No, the triathlon is based on a race in the early-1900s in France that consisted of running, cycling, and canoeing. Considering all of the recent deaths while swimming, maybe it is time to honor tradition and put these people back in canoes. Or maybe we should no longer combine modes of transportation? Swim, bike, or run. Pick one!

## Bodybuilding Contests

If you ever get the urge to attend a sadomasochistic, maladaptive freak show, spend an afternoon at a bodybuilding contest. You will witness exactly where evolution left off and see Neanderthal men in thongs, shaved down, oiled up, and striking strange poses to loud music. Poses include the front double biceps, rear lat spread, and your favorite side triceps. Then you polish off the competition with a crab most muscular pose!

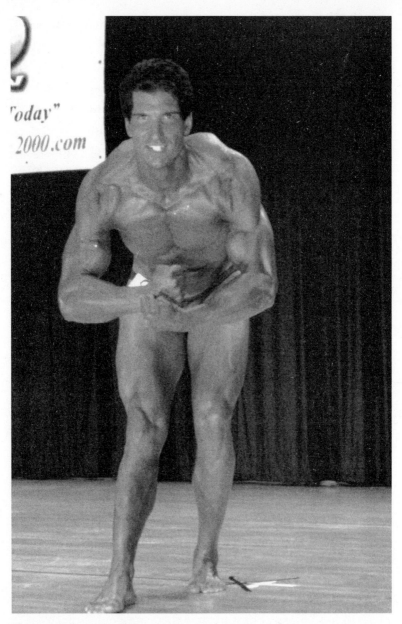

*Showing my most muscular pose to anyone who cares.*

The only difference between a bodybuilding contest and a beauty pageant is that the bodybuilders don't have to speak. Sure, there are a few exceptions to the "meatheaded shitstack" stereotype, but for the vast majority, the farther away they are from a microphone, the better. Bodybuilding is and always will be a sport for insecure baboons. The muscle presents itself as character armor shielding gaping insecurities and a self-esteem the size of a quark.

Since 1999, I have competed naturally in 15 bodybuilding competitions and won three titles. The overriding question I hear is why? What brings someone to step on stage and compete for Best in Show? Essentially, we are dogs that voluntarily chose this medium, unlike the schnauzer that is dragged there by their neurotic owner. I am in the minuscule minority of competitive bodybuilders who have never used steroids. In fact, natural bodybuilding is the ultimate oxymoron. These bizarre events test for steroids by using a polygraph test, also known as a lie detector. They wrap your finger with wires and then try to stump you. "Is your name Andrew Ginsburg?" Yes. "Have you ever lied to get someone else in trouble?" Yes. "Have you ever cheated on an important exam?" Yes. "Have you ever stolen something from a good friend ?" Yes. "Have you ever taken steroids?" No. "Thank you, you passed." Passed? I'm a bad person! I'm going to rot in hell!

Since we know that a lie detector test has the validity of an astrological horoscope, it is all just a formality. Everybody passes, and everyone pays their 200-dollar entry/drug test fee. And if you win, you get a cheap marble trophy that looks really good in an attic window. Backstage, all of the bodybuilders eat rice cakes, jelly, and grilled chicken to remain ripped to the bone, vascular, and pumped. But they drink no water! Nope, water makes you look slightly less ripped, and we can't have that. Then another bodybuilder looks at you and says, "Yo man, that water is gonna taste so good afterwards." Yes, these are all grown men, including some who even went to college. It gets worse—since the lights are bright and white people are pale, we have to paint ourselves brown to look darker and display maximum muscularity.

After you compete against the other idiots in your weight class, you leave for a few hours and then return that night for the finals. This is the glorious portion of the show when the bodybuilders pose to music. Over the years, I have posed to such songs as "Smooth Criminal," "Another Brick in the Wall," and "Rock You Like a Hurricane." And yes, my parents are incredibly proud of me. Once the show is over, you thank the judges and ask them for feedback. They tell you to work on your back, calves, and hamstrings, and then you leave and have a pizza. It's primitive, incredibly weird, and what I do for fun.

# CHAPTER 6
# Faster Phones, Slower Bodies

**THE SOCIAL MEDIA TRAP**

Though technology has enhanced our lives in many ways, it has also made us lazier than at any other point in history. From the comfort of our own home, we can order dinner, clothing, and furniture, and watch any movie at any time without ever having to leave the couch. We can find out the maiden name of Kelly Clarkson's grandmother in a matter of seconds and pull up 50 different recipes for quiche with a few clicks of the keyboard. The only time that we absolutely must rise from our seat is to use the bathroom and answer the door for the delivery guy. With convenience and comfort as the new norm, why would anyone willingly want to expend energy and leave the house to do something as archaic as exercise? Because our body has not changed at the same pace as technology and until a computer chip is inserted into our frontal lobe causing us to exercise and make healthy food choices, we will struggle with our weight and die prematurely. Being overweight raises the risk of heart disease by 32 percent, and a stroke by 24 percent. Furthermore, obesity is now the second-leading cause of cancer after smoking. So don't tell me that you don't have time to work out. Your time depends on working out!

When we are not shopping online, we spend countless hours on social media trolling and posting, tweeting and retweeting, commenting and liking. According to a frightening report by Common Sense Media, a nonprofit focused on helping children, teens in the United States spend on average nine hours a day on media.[1] That's more than they sleep! They also check their favorite social media sites up to 100 times a day. No wonder they don't exercise; they hardly ever move! For adults, the picture is not as dreary yet still miles away from ideal. A recent article in the *New York Times* reported that adults on average spend 50 minutes a day on Facebook.[2] That may not sound so bad, but when you add that complete waste of time on top of important responsibilities such as work and family, you are left with little time to exercise. By simply reducing time on social media, going to the gym becomes much more plausible.

## WHAT'S THE RUSH?

In our Amazon Prime same-day-delivery microcosm, we expect everything immediately and have no interest in delayed gratification. Unfortunately, when it comes to losing weight and building muscle, results are not linear. You will not continue to lose two pounds a week and an inch off of your waist for the next two years. Most likely, you will make strides in the first two or three months and then hit a plateau. Too often, people reach this point, become frustrated, and throw in the towel.

Motivation is crucial to fitness success, which is why one must have realistic expectations. You don't start a job at an entry-level position and expect to be the CEO in a few months, just as you don't take one Spanish class and walk out speaking fluently. Yet for some reason, we demand our weight loss fast— much faster, in fact, than the time it took for the weight gain to take place. We expect to lose twenty pounds in two weeks, even though it took six months to gain that same amount.

These overly ambitious expectations are created by the false advertising on magazine covers and supplement ads. People believe the hype when they read, "Lose ten pounds in ten days!" Wow, do I have to chop off my head to do it? Then there are the ads that proclaim, "Gain two inches on your chest!" Am I getting implants? Obviously, these claims are ridiculous, but if the headline were to read, "Lose ten pounds in three months," then that magazine would be left on the rack. Another common error is when the novice lifter buys a magazine and starts doing Mr. Olympia's chest workout. After two months of heaving around heavy weights for endless sets, his pecs have not grown, and he has injured his rotator cuff. His body was not ready for Mr. Olympia's chest workout, but he didn't know that. What is this rush for overnight fitness? Exercise is a lifestyle, not a crash course. Just once, instead of "I need to lose ten pounds in two weeks," I would love to hear, "I want to be healthy for the rest of my life."

## PUMPING IRON: THE YOGA OF THE WEST

In India, yoga is the physical discipline that is pursued for personal growth, while the Chinese and Japanese prefer Martial Arts. Here in the United States, we do not have an established fitness regime to follow. While obesity levels and prescription pill use increases, we are in desperate need of a healthy vice that points us toward happiness. The most popular form of exercise in this country is walking, followed by running, but neither help to shape a physique. With our 8-second, 140-character attention span and obsession with physical appearance, lifting weights is undoubtedly the perfect fit for us.

While yoga dates back 5,000 years to Northern India, body-building has only been around about a hundred years. It allows for "selfies," Justin Bieber music, and an eternal stare into the mirror. While yogic scriptures can be found in the *Bhagavad-Gita* with deep Hindu roots, lifting weights is not a secular activity, nor is it performed in silence. Yoga focuses on the extension of the muscle, while lifting weights combines both the extension and the contraction. A typical yoga class lasts anywhere from an hour to ninety minutes, while an intense weight workout can be accomplished in thirty minutes, leaving extra time to boast about it on Instagram. By lifting weights, you employ the same discipline as yoga but get to play the role of sculptor and shape your physique.

Weight training is also the most effective form of exercise to lose weight and burn fat because of the elevated metabolism that lasts for many hours after the workout has ended. In a recent study by M.D. Schuenke in the *Journal of Applied Physiology,* seven healthy men were put through a 31-minute workout consisting of four circuits of bench presses, squats, and power cleans doing 10 reps per set and showed an elevated metabolism for well over 16 hours after the workout had ended.[3] This exceeds the 14-hour elevation from a similar study in *Medicine and Science in Sports and Exercise* that monitored a 45-minute workout of intense biking.

## LADIES AND THEIR FEAR OF BIG MUSCLES

Nearly every woman that I have ever trained has expressed the same concern during our first workout together: "I don't want big muscles." This fear has kept many women out of a weight room and glued to a yoga mat or stationary bike. If you're a woman who is worried that pumping iron is going to turn you into The Incredible Hulkette, I have good news for you: it is not going to. You are not going to build huge muscles because you don't have enough testosterone, nor are you going to train with heavy enough weights to build twenty-inch guns. You will, however, build beautiful, shapely muscles that enhance your physique and make you appear even more feminine. Understand that men have about 10 times as much testosterone as you do and still struggle to add muscle size[4] (this is also why we are such assholes, but that is a whole different story). Approach weight training like it's a brand of makeup at Sephora that brings out your best features and hides the weaker ones. By adding and subtracting to certain areas of the your body, you will create the figure that you desire. Studies have also shown that older women who lift weights suffer fewer bone fractures and display better bone quality than the ones who don't.

By lifting weights, you will burn more calories and fat, look better in clothes, and improve your quality of life.

## SHINY MACHINES, FEWER RESULTS

Unfortunately, technology has not ignored the fitness world and has succeeded in producing cardio equipment and weight machines that are easier and more comfy than ever. These high-tech, chrome machines with a fixed design take all the creativity out of performing an exercise and force you to do it only one way. Far superior are free weights because they grant you versatility in range of motion and accommodate any nuance on the exercise. They also require far more energy than their shiny, padded machine counterpart on which you could fall asleep. In reality, you would probably get more out of lifting the machine itself than doing the exercise that it is meant for.

# PART II

# INTRODUCTION

There are three components to getting into great shape: Exercise, nutrition, and relaxation. Leave out any one of the three, and you will not reach your full physical potential. Many think that if they just exercise and eat right, that is enough, but it isn't. The ability and necessity to relax is crucial and includes getting enough sleep, managing stress, and eliciting the relaxation response. The relaxation response is defined as your personal ability to make your body release chemicals and brain signals that make your muscles and organs slow down and increase blood flow to the brain. Transcendental meditation, yoga, and visual imagery are all excellent ways to induce this response. I say "relax" rather than "rest" because a person can still be a ball of stress while lying on the couch. To relax may sound like being lazy, but really it means keeping the mind tranquil. In this country, we ignore this very important component of fitness. The external world trumps the internal one here, while in places like India, it is often the opposite. Relaxation means training your mind the same way you train your body. By reducing stress, you will maximize your workouts and be a happier person.

Some people work out to counter a bad diet, while others eat cleanly so that they don't have to exercise. What a waste! Why not do both parts and create the body that have you always wanted? In life, there are so few things that you can control, so take advantage of the ability to train hard and eat healthy. Then there are people who train hard and eat right but do not get enough sleep at night and walk around exhausted and stressed all day. This is also counterintuitive, since muscle repairs and grows during deep sleep. Finally, there is the couch potato who does none of the three. He doesn't exercise, eats like crap, and lets stress get the best of him. Thankfully, until your life has to come to an end, there is always a chance to improve your physical and mental health. Carl Jung said, "Where the mind goes, the body follows," and I believe the same is true of the reverse. To embark on this holistic approach to being fit, I have designed an easy-to-follow system to include all three components. Each day, I want you to give yourself a grade on all three pieces of the fitness puzzle. For example: If your leg workout or spin class was intense and focused, then give yourself a 100 for exercise. If your nutrition was pretty good but you had a few pieces of bread at dinner, score yourself an 80. If you were stressed the whole day and ran around like a chicken without a head yelling at people and never took the time to calm down and breathe deeply, grade yourself a 60 for relaxation. Now average those three numbers out, and you will see that you scored an 80—not bad, but not your best. By checking in daily, you hold yourself accountable and, more important, become motivated to do your absolute best.

Though this grading system is subjective, be as fair a grader as possible. If you give yourself straight A's when you don't deserve them, the shape of your body will be quick to point that out. The goal is to have all three scores as high and balanced with one another as possible. When you accomplish this, I guarantee that you will love the results.

# CHAPTER 7
# The Fit Foods

"The only way to keep your health is to eat what you don't want, drink what you don't like, and do what you'd rather not."

—Mark Twain

## BONE MEAL BABY

As an infant, I was allergic to nearly every type of food, so my mother had to be creative to ensure that I received the proper nutrients to fuel growth and development. Inventive and artistic, she concocted a drink that she named "The Honey Baba," which consisted of banana, honey, peanut butter, and bone meal. What is bone meal, you ask? It's fertilizer for plants and a mixture of finely ground animal bones and slaughterhouse waste products. In 1979, the year that I was born, bone meal was still being used as a calcium supplement. Then in the early 1980s, researchers discovered that lead and other toxic materials were found in bone meal, and human consumption of

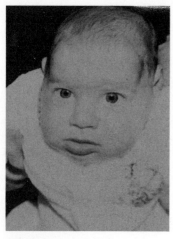
*Baby Beluga*

this concoction declined rapidly. Whether my mother was trying to poison me or just provide me with calcium, I will never know. For sanity's sake, I conveniently choose the latter to protect and preserve my self-esteem. Though the mixture was unorthodox, I now stand 6'3", 215 pounds and have never broken a bone in my life. Maybe bone meal should be brought back to the American diet? Well, maybe not. After years of trial and error, the following are my favorite foods and beverages for building muscle and staying lean—even for someone with a weak stomach.

## FOODS
### Chicken

My relationship with chicken would best be characterized as intimate. For the past ten years, I've eaten a pound a day of high-quality, grade-A boneless, skinless chicken breast and have enjoyed every second of it. Do the math, and you'll see I've wiped out families. To chicken, I'm worse than Stalin. To farmers, I'm a dear friend. Chickens live 5–11 years, take 40 minutes to bake, and are easy for the stomach to digest. The younger they're slaughtered, the more delicious they taste. It's important to recognize that skin has all of the fat, so make sure you take it off, throw it away, and then load up on the white meat. Chicken is a great source of protein, niacin, and selenium. And really, where would we be today without selenium? Exactly.

But not all forms of chicken are healthy. Here are a few ways to take a beautiful thing and fuck it up, accordingly:

Chicken nuggets: In the 1950s, Cornell professor Robert C. Baker came up with the brilliant idea to deep fry chicken in vegetable oil and make everyone around him fat. Six chicken nuggets have 320 calories, 20 grams of fat, and clog up your arteries. Thanks, Bob.

Dark meat: 256 calories per serving, 26 grams of protein, 16 grams of fat (more fat than mayo).

Generals Tso's Chicken: Delicious, filling, and the second worst thing you can possibly eat behind fettuccine Alfredo. 650 calories, 23 grams of fat, and 1,980 mg of sodium. If you eat enough of this dish, you'll look just like the Buddha (the happy, fat one with the big smile, not the fit one under the bodhi tree).

On the other hand, here's how you should eat your chicken.

A 4-ounce serving of boneless, skinless chicken breast has 187 calories, 35 grams of protein, and only 4 grams of fat. Find me a better food for building muscle and staying lean, and I'll show you a chicken dressed up in disguise.

## Salmon

Without salmon, Jews would only put cream cheese on their bagels, sushi restaurants would go bankrupt, and bears, beavers, and otters would starve to death. On a lesser note, without the pink fish, the Canadian economy would collapse. Loaded with protein and the magical omega-3 fatty acids, salmon is one of the healthiest foods you can eat. And if you're an alarmist who worries about mercury content in your food, fear not! Salmon is relatively low in mercury when compared to tuna, bass, and swordfish. Even if you don't like the taste, eat it for your mood! Salmon has long been called a "feel good food" due to its high content of the omega-3 fatty acid docosahexaenoic acid (DHA) that supports brain development and helps fight depression. Salmon benefits the eyes and heart, and even helps you sleep, thanks to its high dosage of tryptophan. The only downside of salmon is the high price and horrible stench it creates when you cook it. To keep your house from smelling like a fish market in Chinatown, wrap up the salmon in tin foil with some lemon slices when you bake it in the oven. Since fish deteriorates fast, make sure you cook it within 24 hours of buying it.

**Eggs**
Fifty years ago, everyone ate the egg yolk and nobody was fat. Now, nobody eats the yolk and everybody is fat. And we eat the part of the egg that tastes like shit! Let's face it, when compared to a traditional yolk-filled omelette, the egg white omelette tastes like crap. To counter the insipid egg white, people add cheese to make it taste better. So, basically you've taken out the fatty yolk and replaced it with fatty cheese. How American of you! Slandered, persecuted, and demonized, the egg yolk is under constant attack because it contains cholesterol. Yes, the yolk also contains virtually all of the vitamins and minerals and half of the egg's protein. Nutrition "experts" contend that by consuming the cholesterol in egg yolks, a person will raise their serum cholesterol levels and increase their risk for arteriosclerosis. While yolks do contain cholesterol, research has found that unless you have a predisposition for high cholesterol levels, eating a yolk or two a day will not adversely affect you. In fact, the University of Connecticut has extensively studied the effects of eggs on cholesterol levels. These controlled studies

have shown that when people consume three to four eggs per day, with the yolk, virtually everyone experiences either no change or beneficial changes in their cholesterol.[1]

I recently read an article in a newspaper that said that eating egg yolks is almost as bad as smoking. Really? Who was the last person who ate an eggs Benedict and developed throat polyps? Or had so many egg yolks that he needed an iron lung? How many mothers gave birth to three-pound infants because they had three eggs over easy? That's right, none. Eat the yolk, cut out the cheese, and enjoy your eggs!

## Oatmeal

If you want to lose weight, lower your cholesterol, and stay fuller for longer, you should eat oatmeal every day for breakfast. The magic mush is high in soluble fiber and is a slow-burning carbohydrate that provides energy for 2-3 hours after eating it. Oatmeal may even help you live longer! In a Harvard University study, researchers discovered that those who ate whole grains equivalent to a bowl of oatmeal a day reduced their risk of premature death by 9 percent and their risk of dying of heart disease by 15 percent.[2]

I know I may sound like an oatmeal commercial, and that is my intention. Because of the slow digestion process, try to wait at least 90 minutes after eating it to go to the gym. If you don't have the luxury of 90 minutes, have a banana twenty minutes before your workout and then have a bowl of oatmeal afterwards. If you find oatmeal bland, spice it up with blueberries, banana, walnuts, or honey. And if you want to treat yourself to something delicious, mix a tablespoon of peanut butter with a tablespoon of honey into your oatmeal, and it will taste like dessert.

## Sweet Potato

Sweet potatoes receive one day of love—on Thanksgiving—and are forgotten about the rest of the year. It's like ignoring your girlfriend every day except for Valentine's Day and then smothering her with gifts. According to the Center of Science in the Public Interest, the sweet potato ranked highest in nutritional value of any vegetable.[3] That's right, number one! It beat out spinach, broccoli, and even defeated the almighty kale. Loaded with vitamins A, C, D, B6, as well as potassium, magnesium, and dietary fiber, the sweet potato tastes too good to be so healthy. When baked, it creates a soothing aroma better than any scented candle and is extremely easy to prepare. Just preheat your oven to 350 degrees F. Wash the sweet potato and then puncture it with a knife across the top. Place it on a baking sheet, sprinkle on some cinnamon, and depending on thickness, bake anywhere from 45 to 70 minutes.

## Avocado

This low-carb fruit is extremely high in potassium and a godsend in taste and texture. Though 77 percent of the calories in an avocado come from fat, the majority of the fat comes from oleic acid, an omega-9 fatty acid that is the main component of olive oil and has been shown to lower cholesterol levels.[4] An avocado is high in fiber and antioxidants like lutein and zeaxanthin, both of which are important for eye health. Famous for its lead role in guacamole, avocado works wonders in salads, sushi, and as a substitute for mayonnaise.

## Tuna Fish

Tuna fish swim up to 55 mph and taste really good when mixed with mayonnaise. I was raised on this fine delicacy at least three nights a week. My mom would throw three cans of tuna fish into a large bowl, plus a couple of spoonfuls of mayonnaise, and dinner was served. My sisters and I would take turns mashing the tuna and mixing the mayo. On special occasions, when we behaved ourselves, my mom would chop up a Granny Smith apple and throw it in the bowl along with the tuna fish and mayo. She would say that fish is good for your eyes, and my dad would say it's brain food. They were both right. It's also good for your skin, mood, and heart. A can of tuna fish provides 26 grams of protein. To make tuna salad healthier, eat Hellmann's Light Mayo. Unlike other low-fat substitutes, Hellmann's Light actually tastes like mayo. And if you want to make your tuna fish even healthier, use avocado instead of mayo. Remember to buy albacore tuna fish packed in water, not oil, and that chunk light tuna is disgusting.

Here are a few ways to take a healthy fish and ruin it:
- Tuna Casserole (cheese, creamed soup, and mayo).
- Using real mayo in excess.

**Apple**
We all know that apples "keep the doctor away," but specifically, they prevent heart disease, cancer, type 2 diabetes, stroke, and Alzheimer's disease, and help lower cholesterol. Loaded with vitamin C, antioxidants, and fiber, apples are a great snack that satisfy a sweet tooth and should be consumed daily. Don't worry about eating the right kind of apple, because they all share similar properties. Whether you prefer Honey Crisp, Granny Smith, Red Delicious, or Fuji, you will still reap the benefits of the so-called "miracle food." Since apples do contain fructose, set a two-apples-a-day limit to prevent weight gain.

## Banana

They are delicious, and the most popular fruit in the United States. The beauty of bananas lies in quick energy. If you are in a rush to get to the gym and haven't eaten anything, a banana is the perfect food choice. Studies have shown that those who eat bananas 4–6 times a week are almost 50 percent less likely to develop kidney disease, compared to people who don't eat bananas.[5] An excellent source of vitamin B6 and potassium, bananas should be a daily part of your diet. I mix a banana in my oatmeal and then blend one in my protein shake following a workout.

## Blueberry

Trailing only strawberries in popularity among berries, blueberries are the healthiest berry in the world because they are highest in antioxidants and loaded with vitamin C, vitamin K, and manganese. Studies have shown blueberries to help memory, vision, and cardiovascular health. Rather than use a muffin as a gateway to blueberries, put them in your oatmeal and increase the taste tenfold.

## White Rice

One question I hear frequently that disgusts me more and more each time is "Do you have brown rice sushi?" "No, they don't have brown rice sushi. Sushi is made with white rice! Eat it like a normal Japanese person!" Besides removing any semblance of taste, brown rice sushi is no healthier than real sushi. In fact, brown rice is harder to digest than white rice due to the high fiber content from the bran and germ that gives it that brown color. The difference in calories, carbohydrates, and protein between the two are negligible, and brown rice contains phytic acid, whereas white rice is pure starch.

Starch has been vilified like the egg yolk even though our bodies run on glucose as their primary energy source. Now that we've knocked brown rice off its fibrous pedestal, I also want to tell you that long-grain versus short-grain rice is another wasteful comparison. They are both starch, and the difference between the two is, once again, minuscule. Because white rice is high on the glycemic index and raises blood sugar quickly, it is best to eat immediately after a workout to offset the low blood sugar caused from intense exercise. Billions of people around the world eat a diet high in white rice and incidentally, have long life expectancies. The people of Okinawa and Japan smoke cigarettes, engorge white rice, and live forever. They do not eat brown rice, nor are they obese. Of course, if you prefer the taste of brown rice to white rice, then by all means, cook it at home and eat it. Just don't ask for brown rice when you're out for sushi!

## Sushi

What is it about these fragments of raw fish that enable sushi restaurants to charge an arm and a leg for a gill and a fin? Take a piece of raw fish, stick it on a bed of rice, and voilà, you've got five bucks in your pocket. I could get two cans of tuna for that price with twice the amount of protein. So why does sushi cost more than a can of tuna? The same reason fancy clothes cost more: because it's elegant to look at. They line the sushi up on a wooden block and seduce you with the colors—green avocado, red tuna, orange salmon, all wrapped up around some white rice and green cucumber. Throw in some wasabi, soy sauce, and ginger, and you have yourself a vibrant, kaleidoscopic feast. Sushi first became popular in the United States in the late 1960s, when a sushi chef created the California roll, replacing tuna with avocado and putting the seaweed on the inside so Americans did not have to bite directly into it. Sushi is high in protein, carbs, and has the holy grail of fats—the cherished, revered omega-3. A few suggestions to keep sushi a healthy meal and not a shitfest:

1. Stick to pieces of sushi or sashimi, specifically yellowtail, salmon, tuna, and mackerel. Eel will turn you into a whale, as will too many "special" rolls. Six pieces of sushi or sashimi, one roll, and a salad is a healthy meal.
2. Stay away from anything with an American city in the name: Philadelphia rolls and Boston rolls are both high in fat and calories, while rolls named after states, such as Alaskan rolls and California rolls, are better choices.
3. Go easy on the spicy mayo.
4. Don't ask for a fork.

**Spinach**

During the Great Depression, the television show "Popeye the Sailor" premiered and saved the dying spinach industry by boosting consumption by 33 percent.[6] People saw the great strength that Popeye gained from spinach and went out to the supermarket to reap the reward. It would be one of the only times in history that television influenced the public to eat healthy. The leafy green is loaded with potassium, magnesium, and vitamin K. From your skin to your bones and your hair to your heart, spinach offers vitamins and minerals that prevent diseases such as diabetes and certain types of cancer. Spinach is also much easier to digest than broccoli or cauliflower. Boiled, sautéed, or eaten raw, spinach should be a part of your diet.

## Broccoli

Broccoli is and always will be the Don Corleone of the cabbage family. These little green flowers are loaded with vitamin C and D, as well as beta-carotene, and have been shown to reduce risk of heart disease and certain cancers. Broccoli contains something called sulforaphane, which may help combat prostate, liver, lung, bladder, skin, and stomach cancer. The healthiest way to cook broccoli is to boil it. But be careful not to overindulge at dinner, or your family will suffer the foul-smelling consequences.

## Walnut

The walnut is the nut highest in omega-3 fatty acids and by just eating 14 halves a day, you increase the health of your heart, hair, and skin, and may even reduce depression. The walnut also has strong anti-inflammatory effects and helps lower cholesterol. Research has shown walnuts to assist in brain function, especially in old age, and possibly ward off neurological disorders such as Alzheimer's disease.[7] The delicious taste works well in oatmeal and salads, or eaten alone.

## BEVERAGES
### Water

In this country, if a beverage doesn't leave you drunk or caffeinated, Americans have little to no use for it. As the largest consumer in the world of beer and soda, the US has neglected water, whereas water spin-offs have reigned supreme. Vitaminwater bears the name, but is really just a fruity version of Coke that is loaded with sugar and not as "healthy" as the label leads you to believe. For a fluid that covers 70 percent of the Earth, makes up 60 percent of your body, and keeps you from smelling like a foot, it makes sense to drink the pure version over the "enhanced" sugary one. Each morning, everyone should wake up and immediately chug 16 ounces of water to jump-start your brain and body. Breakfast is always referred to as the most important meal of the day because you haven't eaten in 7–10 hours. Well, you also have not drunk anything over that time and probably made some trips to the bathroom during the night. You may swear by coffee to wake you up, but you also need water to hydrate you. So, from now on, double-fist your coffee with a large glass of water. And then when you're done with that, have another glass.

Water aids in digestion, flushes out toxins, lubricates the joints, and keeps your memory sharp. The Institute of Medicine says women need around 90 ounces a day and men need about 125 ounces daily.[8] If you're an athlete sweating all day long, you need even more. Water is absolutely essential to the human body's survival. A person can live for about a month without food, but only about a week without water. Since the average American falls a quart short of the recommended daily water intake, it is not surprising that the most common cause of daytime fatigue is dehydration. In a country that sells 109 brands of bottled water, the fact that we're dehydrated is pretty sad.

Within the billion-dollar bottled water industry, Smart water and Fiji have the prettiest bottles, while Aquafina and Evian have the ugliest. Personally, I drink a gallon a day of New York City's finest tap water. In fact, a study conducted by microbiologist Aaron Margolin of the University of New Hampshire found that there was no difference between the New York City tap water and the bottled waters that were evaluated, in terms of their chemical make-up.[9] The key to adequate water consumption is to drink all day long, with the majority of your intake between meals. Too much water during meals can interfere with digestion. In particular, too much cold water during meals can slow digestion and may cause cramping in sensitive individuals. The more water you drink between meals, the less likely you are to overeat, since your stomach is already full of water.

## Coffee

Is coffee a friend or a foe? I say friend. I say best friend. I say friend who helps you move. 108 million Americans agree with me. In fact, the Sufis of Yemen first enjoyed the soothing aroma, taste, and caffeine spike in the midfifteenth century that is still worshipped to this day. Of course, there is always that vegan yogi who will approach you at a coffee shop and say, "You should really switch to tea." Yeah, well you should really mind your own business. Tea is what you drink when you're sick. Coffee is what you drink when you want to wake up. This may sound biased, and that's because it is. Personally, I like a little bias in my coffee.

Harvard researchers say drinking coffee lowers the risk of Parkinson's disease, colon cancer, and type 2 diabetes.[10] According to scientists at Vanderbilt University's Institute for Coffee Studies (yes, it exists, I checked), research shows coffee to be far healthier than it is harmful.[11] The average 8-ounce cup of coffee has 85 mg of caffeine. An Excedrin has 120mg and a Diet Coke 45 mg. Coffee not only prevents headaches but has been linked directly to stronger muscle contractions. Finally, it makes you more alert and enhances concentration, a great counter to our country's short attention span. Because caffeine can keep you up at night, I would recommend having your last cup of coffee no later than 2 p.m.

## Alcohol

In a city full of drunks, the question I get asked most by my clients is "What should I drink when I go out?" After I say "water" and they roll their eyes, I tell them to drink red wine. Not white wine, but red. White wine lacks the antioxidants that the biblical red wine procures. The average glass of red has 120 calories and is loaded with flavonoids and nonflavonoids, those magical antioxidants that reduce blood clots and lower cholesterol in rats. Since humans are an exact replica of rats, one must assume that we share the same benefits. Pick a red like merlot, cabernet, malbec, or pinot noir because it has much less residual sugar than a sweet one.

Now, if you don't like red wine, order vodka or whiskey. James Bond drinks nothing but martinis, and he's always ripped. Both vodka and whiskey are about 100 calories (one shot). If you prefer beer, choose Guinness. Made from more grains than lager, Guinness actually has antioxidant properties similar to red wine. Like rats and humans, Guinness and red wine are Siamese twins.

Now, if you're looking to destroy any semblance of muscular definition and add girth to your frame, opt for a piña colada, Scorpion Bowl, margarita, Long Island iced tea, or Jack and Coke. And if cardiac arrest is what you seek, a Red Bull with vodka has your name written all over it. The idiocy of mixing a stimulant and a depressant will always baffle me.

Like a comedy club, opt for the two-drink minimum (and maximum). Any more than two drinks, and you'll wake up fatter, plus you'll feel the need to eat a bacon, egg, and cheese sandwich to nurse the hangover. The greasy sandwich will line your stomach and slow down the absorption of alcohol, but it will not help your waistline.

## SUPPLEMENTS

The use of dietary supplements can be a great way to maximize gains or a quick way to throw away money. They can even be hazardous to your health. Supplements are meant as just that—something you add to something else to enhance it, not replace it. That something else is food, the best delivery service of nutrients to your body. Today, most people who exercise use at least some form of supplementation. Protein shakes and preworkout cocktails have become the norm, as gym members walk around the weight room with shaker bottles containing a strange blue liquid designed to fuel their workout. But what's really in this strange blue liquid? Not even the sales guy in the polo shirt at the health food store can tell you. He can read the label and sell it, but he cannot possibly know the contents, since supplements do not require FDA-approval to be sold in stores. According to a recent *New York Times* article, "'Of about 55,000 supplements that are sold in the United States, only 170—about 0.3 percent—have been studied closely enough to determine their common side effects,' said Dr. Paul A. Offit, the chief of infectious diseases at the Children's Hospital of Philadelphia and an expert on dietary supplements."[12] Free of government regulation, companies can sell you muscle mass and fat loss at a high price in the form of a mystery powder. It could be sugar or it could be cocaine. Or it could be 100 percent whey protein, like the label says. And since the majority of supplements try their best to mimic the effects of steroids to some degree, there is a decent chance that your anabolic agent or thermogenic aid could be dangerous. If you choose to use supplements, buy a reputable brand of protein powder and not the one called "Big Eddie's Anabolic Drink." For years, I have used IsoPure Zero Carb Whey Protein Isolate by Nature's Valley and had good results. Protein bars, on the other hand, made me fat. They taste like "Snickers" for a reason, and I'd end up eating too many of them. When I tried the hugely popular creatine monohydrate, I felt bloated and gross and quickly stopped taking it. There are three supplements that I believe in:

1. **Whey Protein Isolate** – Has the highest bioavailability of any protein powder, which means that your body can absorb and digest whey better than any other source.
2. **Branched-Chain Amino Acids (BCAAs)** – Amino acids are the building blocks of protein and facilitate muscle growth.
3. **Multivitamin** – I take this as an insurance policy to make sure that I'm getting all of the vitamins and minerals that my body needs.

Don't waste your money and risk your health on the latest "cutting edge" supplement. Instead, go to the grocery store and buy some chicken and oatmeal.

# CHAPTER 8
# The One-Third Diet

"Pure reason avoids extremes, and requires one to be wise in moderation."

—Molière

The best way that I have found to build muscle and stay lean is to consume a diet that consists of one-third protein, one-third carbohydrates, and one-third fat. Extreme ratios of protein to carbs to fat have become the norm, so a call back to balance is long overdue. A legendary pro bodybuilder and mentor, Phil Hernon, introduced this diet to me, and it has provided me with the energy and nutrients to get in the best shape of my life. Before I forget, we better name the diet, or there will be mayhem in the streets. Since each macronutrient represents a third of all calories, "The One-Third Diet" seems the logical choice.

This diet is extremely easy to follow. Each meal will consist of approximately 360 calories and is made up of 30 grams of protein,

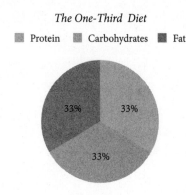

*The One-Third Diet*

■ Protein   ■ Carbohydrates   ■ Fat

33%   33%   33%

30 grams of carbs, and 13 grams of fat. Why are there more grams of protein and carbs than fat? Because a gram of protein and carbohydrates each has four calories while a gram of fat has nine. The more muscle you carry, the more calories you will need, so feel free to increase the calories of each meal. If your goal is to build muscle mass, I would recommend eating 40 grams of protein, 40 grams of carbs, and 18 grams of fat at each meal, for a total of 480 calories. If you are trying to lose weight and find that a one-third ratio at each meal is not working for you, lower the calories and cycle carbohydrates so that your biggest serving is at breakfast, second largest at lunch, and smallest portion at dinner. To keep daily totals of nutrients to a ⅓ market share, you would do the opposite for protein and have your smallest portion at breakfast, medium size at lunch, and largest at dinner. Now, let's have a look at each macronutrient.

## CARBS

The word "carbs" (no one says "carbohydrate," ever) has become synonymous with "evil" because of a doctor named Atkins and his now-defunct church that preached carbs as the devil. Carbs are not the devil! Processed food is the devil. Refined sugar is the devil. Bad timing is the devil. Carbs provide our muscles with energy and are essential for brain function. In a 2009 study, researchers found that people on a high-fat, low-carb diet for a year had more anger, anxiety, and depression than people on a low-fat, high-carb diet.[1] When the carb level is kept low, the body uses fat as its energy source. Though this may sound desirable, fat is nowhere near as efficient an energy source as carbs, and the result is often a feeling of fatigue. Brain cells function best on glucose but cannot run on fats directly, so ketones are released into the blood, and the brain generates them into energy.[2] When elevated levels of ketone bodies are in the blood and are being used as energy, you are in a state of ketosis, the goal of the highly popular ketogenic diet. While many people may thrive on a ketogenic diet, I have always felt weak, tired, and irritable when I dropped my carbs too low. Rather than restrict carbs completely, they make up one third of my total calories, which is still low compared to the 45 to 60 percent recommendation by the Dietary Guidelines For Americans.

In 1981, Dr. David Jenkins at the University of Toronto developed the Glycemic Index (GI) to display the speed at which certain foods raise blood sugar levels. The healthiest carbs are the ones that are low GI foods and raise blood glucose levels slowly, sustaining energy for a longer period. If blood sugar spikes too quickly, it causes insulin overload, which can lead to weight gain. You cannot burn fat while maintaining a high insulin level. Insulin is a hormone that causes your body's cells to take glucose (sugar) and store it in the liver to be used as energy. However when insulin is low, the body can use fat as energy, which is the goal when trying to get lean. If blood sugar levels remain elevated, it can be toxic and cause heart disease, Type 2 Diabetes, and kidney failure. The only time high GI foods are beneficial is postworkout to offset the hypoglycemia caused by intense exercise.

Oatmeal, brown rice, and sweet potatoes are superhealthy carbs and low GI foods that provide energy and loads of vitamins and minerals. High GI foods are white bread, bagels, baked potatoes, pasta, candy, soft drinks, cereals loaded with

| Glycemic Index | | |
|---|---|---|
| Low Glycemic Foods List 0-55 (Good) | Medium Glycemic Foods List 56-70 (Okay) | High Glycemic Foods List 70+ (Bad) |
| Tomatoes 15 | White Rice 56 | Watermelon 72 |
| Peas 22 | Pita Bread 57 | Bagel 72 |
| Grapefruit 25 | Bran Muffin 60 | Honey 73 |
| Low-fat Yogurt 33 | Ice Cream 61 | Doughnuts 75 |
| Apple 36 | Raisins 64 | French Fries 76 |
| Banana 53 | Couscous 65 | White Bread 79 |
| Sweet Potato 54 | Pineapple 66 | Pretzels 81 |
| Oatmeal 55 | Whole Wheat Bread 68 | Baked Potato 85 |

sugar, pretzels, and chips. If you have to eat bread, make sure it is whole grain, and if you like pasta, well, you have good taste.

Here are the healthiest ways to eat approximately 30 grams of carbohydrates:

1 banana: 27 grams of carbohydrates

1 serving of oatmeal: 27 grams of carbohydrates

1 apple: 25 grams of carbohydrates

1 medium sweet potato: 25 grams of carbohydrate

½ cup white or brown rice: 23 grams of carbohydrates

2 slices of rye or whole wheat bread: 24 grams of carbohydrates

## PROTEIN
Protein builds and repairs muscle tissue, helps produce hormones and enzymes, and composes your luxurious, flowing head of hair and perfectly manicured finger nails. If carbs are the most chastised macronutrient, protein is the most revered. Protein sources should come from chicken, fish, eggs, turkey, lean meat, and protein shakes. If you are a vegan or vegetarian, protein should come from soy and quinoa because they

contain all nine of the essential amino acids. You can also combine plant sources (i.e., soy products, quinoa, brown rice and beans, hummus and pita, tofu, lentils, etc.) to get all the amino acids. Of the 20 amino acids in your body's proteins, nine are essential to your diet because your cells cannot manufacture them: histidine, isoleucine, leucine, lysine, methionine, phenylalanine, threonine, tryptophan, and valine.

The recommended daily allowance for protein is 0.36 grams per pound of body weight, which means a 140-pound woman needs approximately 53 grams of protein. The more you exercise, the more protein you require. In fact, the American College of Sports Medicine recommends that to increase muscle mass through exercise, you need to consume 0.5 to 0.8 grams of protein per pound of body weight.[3] I have experienced my best results by eating 1 gram of protein per pound of body weight while on an intense five-day-a-week workout regimen. Since each person's body and metabolism is unique, it is important to observe how you feel and how your muscles respond to different amounts of protein. Some may require up to a gram per pound of body weight to build muscle, while others can make gains on far less. Here are some healthy ways to eat approximately 30 grams of protein:

4 oz of chicken breast: 31 grams of protein

5 oz of salmon: 28 grams of protein

4 oz of steak: 28 grams of protein

4 eggs: 24 grams of protein

8 egg whites: 29 grams of protein (but eat the yolk!)

1 can of tuna fish: 23 grams of protein

4 oz ground turkey: 30 grams of protein

3 cups of quinoa: 24 grams of protein

1 scoop of Isopure Whey Protein: 25 grams of protein

100 almonds: 25 grams of protein (also 700 calories!)

## FAT

In the early 1980s, the government saw Americans getting fatter than ever and issued a statement that they should cut down dietary fat to a maximum of 30 percent of their calories. Like good, law-abiding citizens, we put down the cheeseburger and butter and picked up the sugar—lots and lots of sugar! We figured, "Well, it's better than fat, right?" Fast-forward thirty years, and this country is in worse physical shape than it was then. The sugar with which we replaced our fat causes insulin levels to spike, which makes fat loss nearly impossible.

Certain types of fat are not only good for your health, but some such as omega-3 and omega-6 fatty acids are essential. Omega-3 fatty acids help lower cholesterol and blood pressure, alleviate joint pain, boost your mood, and promote healthy skin. The best sources of omega-3 fatty acids are salmon, halibut, mackerel, walnuts, flaxseed, sardines, and egg yolks. Omega-6 fatty acids help brain function, promote healthy hair and skin, maintain bone health, and regulate metabolism. Avocado, olive oil, vegetable oil, sunflower oil, and walnuts are all great sources of omega-6 fatty acid.

Saturated fat is the most unhealthy type of fat because it raises the level of cholesterol in your blood and increases the risk of heart disease and stroke. Foods high in saturated fat include fatty beef, pork, lamb, butter, cheese, and cream. If you are a cheese lover (after all, almost everyone is), provolone and mozzarella are lower in saturated fat than cheddar, American, and Monterey Jack.

Here are the healthiest ways to eat approximately 13 grams of fat:

Half an avocado: 13 grams of fat

4 oz of salmon: 14 grams of fat

20 almonds: 12 grams of fat

1 ½ tablespoons of peanut butter: 12 grams of fat

1 tablespoon of olive oil: 14 grams of fat

2 eggs: 10 grams of fat

1 handful of walnuts: 13 grams of fat

## CALORIES

The average person burns around 15 calories per pound of body weight a day, so at 215 pounds, I have to eat around 3,225 calories to maintain my weight. To lose weight, I should eat 12 calories per pound of body weight, and to gain weight, I require 18 calories per pound. Again, these are all approximations, and only through trial and error will you find the right calorie count to help you lose, gain, or maintain weight. For the record, I have never counted calories and believe that far more important than caloric content are the food choices you make. A bowl of oatmeal is approximately 150 calories, the same as 44 M&Ms. The former is high in fiber and will keep you full for hours, while the latter is pure sugar and will make you even hungrier. One is a blueprint for weight loss and the other, weight gain. If you make healthy food choices consistently, you will not need to count calories. However, if counting calories works for you, it is now easier than ever before with free apps on the iPhone such as "Lose It!" and "MyFitnessPal." Just enter the foods you have eaten, and it will do the rest for you.

## MY FAVORITE RECIPES

When I was growing up, Hellmann's Real Mayonnaise was one of my favorite foods, if you want to call it that. I looked for any excuse to eat it and put it on everything. My favorite concoctions were mayonnaise sandwiches on white bread and white rice with mayo. Of course, I made sure to use generous amounts of mayo for chicken salad, tuna salad, and turkey sandwiches, as well. As I grew older and more health-conscious, I kept mayonnaise in the mix but switched to Hellmann's Light Mayo, which is lower in calories but retains most of the great taste. Even when training for a bodybuilding competition, I kept Hellmann's Light in the mix. Here are some of my favorite recipes.

### Chicken Surprise

Boneless, skinless chicken breasts

Chopped broccoli

White Rice

Avocado

Onion

Low-fat mayo

Bake, broil, or grill the chicken breasts and then cut them into small cubes. Finely chop up the onion and slice the avocado. Mix the three ingredients into a large bowl with the cooked white rice and chopped broccoli and then add one tablespoon of light mayo. Mix it up well and then serve warm. The taste is delicious, and the meal is loaded with protein, carbs, and the "good" fat. Brown rice can be used in place of white rice, but I have always preferred white rice both for taste and ease of digestion.

Note: Chicken surprise can transform into tuna surprise, salmon surprise, or even egg surprise with the use or tuna, salmon, or eggs in place of the chicken.

## Turkey Burgers

2 lb. ground turkey

½ onion (finely chopped)

2 eggs

Salt

Pepper

Mix all of the ingredients together in a bowl, form into patties, and then broil or grill turkey burgers.

## Baked Salmon (That Doesn't Stink Up the Kitchen)

1 lb salmon fillet

2 tablespoons lemon juice

2 tablespoons of olive oil

Sprinkle olive oil and lemon juice on the salmon fillet and then place salmon on a sheet of tin foil oiled side down. Wrap up the salmon by folding the tin foil over so it is completely sealed. Bake for approximately 25 minutes.

## Apple Walnut Tuna Salad

2 cans of albacore tuna in water

1 chopped Granny Smith apple

1 handful of walnuts

1 tablespoon of Hellmann's Light Mayo

Mix the ingredients and serve.

If mayonnaise is my favorite taste, peanut butter is a close second. Here is my favorite protein shake recipe:

**Peanut Butter Delight**

2 scoops of Isopure Zero Carb Whey Protein Powder

1 banana

1 tablespoon of peanut butter

1 tablespoon of honey

Throw ingredients in a blender with lots of ice and half a cup of water or almond milk and blend on high.

## ODE TO TUPPERWARE

Unless you have several hours free each day to cook, you need to become closely acquainted with high-quality, microwave-safe Tupperware. If you consistently have healthy food prepared and ready to eat, you will make better food choices. That is why it is imperative that you prepare your food in bulk. Boil two dozen eggs, bake three pounds of chicken, broil two pounds of fish, and steam lots of green vegetables and then store them away in Tupperware in the refrigerator. When three or four days' worth of food is prepared, staying on course with your diet is easy. It's when you have to venture out into the world and let a restaurant feed you "mystery meals" that unwanted weight piles up. Pack your lunch in Tupperware and bring it to work. And don't skimp on the kind of Tupperware you buy because cheap kinds leak. Splurge on the highest-quality Tupperware and don't just rinse and reuse it each time because a lax cleaning job will not kill the bacteria that hangs out long after your chicken breast has been eaten. Take the time to scrub each piece with soap thoroughly before using it again. If you bring your Tupperware to work, make sure you don't leave it unrefrigerated for too long. Foods such as chicken, eggs, fish, and anything prepared with mayo need to be cooled at or below 40 degrees Fahrenheit. If you leave your food at room temperature for several hours, you risk allowing bacteria to grow and contaminate your food. As soon as your Tupperware is empty, it's time to start cooking again.

---

**TAKEAWAYS**

- Keep your daily total of nutrients to ⅓ protein, ⅓ carbohydrates, and ⅓ fat.
- Take in at least 25 grams of protein at every meal.
- As soon as you wake up, drink 2 glasses (16 ounces) of water.
- The only carbs you should eat at dinner should be in the form of leafy green vegetables.
- Drink the majority of your water in between meals—not during them—so you don't interrupt digestion.
- Never skip breakfast.
- Minimize processed foods and refined sugar. Better yet, eliminate them.
- Only eat when you are hungry, not because it's been two or three hours since your last meal.
- Eat oatmeal every single day for breakfast.
- Dessert is not an option (unless it's a cheat day).

---

# CHAPTER 9
# Training Time

**RISE AND SHINE**

The early bird gets the worm, and the late one starves to death. That is why it is imperative to go to the gym before work, not after. At 6 a.m., there is a solitude and serenity that does not exist later in the day after your boss yells at you, your wife files for divorce, and your parents cut you out of the will. The longer you are awake, the more opportunities people have to use your ears as toilets, piss on your hours, and provide you with a reason to skip the gym. By working out first thing in the morning, you set a positive tone for the day that will leave you focused, energetic, and confident to deal with the demands that lie ahead.

If you are a night owl, the prospect of a 6 a.m. workout is laughable, since it's hard enough to just get up to use the bathroom at that time. Instead, you shlep to the gym after work and wait twenty minutes for a treadmill and another ten for a bench, and settle for a crappy workout. Just get up early and go! Like anything else, you will get used to it. And whether you need coffee, speed, or cocaine to get you out of bed is of no concern. Just get in there and blast! When you work out at night, your body temperature rises and you become more alert, which screws up your sleep cycle. The training stimulates the heart, brain, and muscles, which is the exact opposite of what you want before bed. It's worth getting up early to exercise in order to sleep well at night. Plus, you can burn up to three times as much fat early in the morning because of the empty glycogen stores in your muscles. Another problem with working out at night is that it forces you to eat dinner late, so that not only is there blood in your muscles, but now you're making it rush to your stomach to digest dinner. This causes your body temperature to rise further, which is not conducive to deep sleep. Exercise first thing in the morning, and you'll be in better physical and mental shape for the rest of the day.

## ONE HOUR MAX

When I go to the gym, I have a strict rule that I abide by: once I have been there an hour, I turn around and leave. Whether I spend that time talking to a friend, watching TV, or squatting until I drop, I stick to it. Quite frankly, if you cannot complete a workout in an hour, you are not exerting yourself enough. The majority of people waste far too much time at the gym wandering around, talking, and staring into space. They arrive with no plan and make up the workout as they go along. "Let's see, I'll do a set of crunches on the ab machine and then watch a YouTube video and stare at the chick on the hip abductor. Then I'll slowly walk over to the water fountain, have a drink, and then become mesmerized by the infomercial on TV." It's almost as if one will do anything to avoid the pain and discomfort of exercise.

The other extreme is the gym rat that works out hard for three hours straight. One may assume that with exercise, more means better. Nothing could be further from the truth! A three hour workout will leave you overtrained, frustrated, and injured. The joints and muscles are not made to support three hours of continuous exercise. Like an alcoholic, a gym rat will spend a large portion of their day intoxicating themselves in escapism until their body breaks down, medical bills fly high, and they're left depressed at home on the couch. Just like a bartender cuts off a mean drunk, I think the fitness manager at the gym should remove a compulsive exerciser at the two-hour mark. Muscles don't strengthen at the gym, they break down. So, a three-hour daily workout will actually make your muscles atrophy. The magic takes place at home when you rest, eat, and sleep. Symptoms of overtraining include insomnia, headaches, depression, and injury. I recommend that you take a minimum of one day off from exercise each week and more if your body tells you to. Everyone should hit the gym hard for 45 minutes to an hour and then go home and eat, rest, and recover. You'll look better in the long run and even have time for a social life.

## TWO MAGIC WORDS

The former Ivy League frat boy in the sleeveless, JP Morgan Corporate Challenge t-shirt makes his beeline to the bench press and marks his territory with a plush navy blue towel and an orange Gatorade bottle. He lies down on the bench, knocks out 15 lightning-fast reps with one 45-pound plate on each side of the bar, emphatically racks it, and pops up as the proud victor. Then he checks himself out in the mirror to make sure he still exists and answers a quick e-mail on his iPhone. His next move is to place another 25-pound plate on each side of the bar and then lies down and bounces the bar off his chest ten more times. His chest looks like nothing because he's never trained it before. He thinks he has and doesn't realize that his shoulders and triceps have been doing all of the work. He will do this for the rest of his life and thus will forever maintain an Ivy league brain with a community college physique.

Two words that will change this man's body and workout forever are "stretch" and "contract." That's it! Our friend here does neither, and that is because the banker is not invested in each repetition. To many lifters, a set is defined as moving a weight from point A to point B, fifteen times, as fast as you can. To stretch a muscle properly, you must control the negative part of the motion and do full-range repetitions. By the negative part, I am referring to the eccentric part of the motion where the muscle stretches (for example, when you do a biceps curl and lift the bar to your shoulders, the negative part is when you lower the bar back down). Half-reps build half-muscles, and half-muscles look wholly ridiculous. Instead, take two seconds on the negative part of the movement as you lower the bar down to your chest and then press it up and contract your chest as hard as you possibly can. Do not lock out your elbows at the top of the movement, as that takes tension off of the chest and moves it into the triceps. By stretching and contracting your muscles, you will develop full-muscle bellies with good shape. It's not about swinging a weight from point A to point B fifteen times. The muscle could care less what the poundage is if it's not actually doing the work to lift the weight.

On the other hand, the muscle is obsessed with the contraction throughout the set. When the mind and muscle are connected as one, your body will improve quickly and you will understand what proper training is all about. Now, this is much easier said than done and takes years to learn. For example, when training the back muscles, most people are working out their biceps with little to no back involved. And it makes sense! How often do you contract your back muscles? Hardly ever. Your biceps? All day long. The average person has never been told to pull with their elbows and crunch their shoulder blades together.

Try it today. Cut back on the weight, slow down the reps, and watch your body pump up. Let the masses swing their heavy weights and build up their ego. Separate yourself from the pack and don't worry about what other people are doing.

## DRAW A CIRCLE

To keep constant tension on the muscle being worked, think of each repetition and set of an exercise as a circle that never stops moving. It goes round and round and round until the muscle reaches failure and can no longer perform another repetition. That means not locking out your knees and pausing after each rep of squats and not allowing your arms to come to a complete stop at the bottom part of a biceps curl. Keep the muscles working continuously until they can't go any more.

## INTENSITY

High-intensity workouts are the most effective way to build muscle and burn fat, but the problem is that the word "intensity" is thrown around nearly as much as "core," "organic," and "functional." If you grunt as loudly as you can with each rep and then throw down your weights at the end of a set, it doesn't mean you're intense; it just means you're a jerk. If you are texting or staring into space, it may be less disturbing than the roaring narcissist, but it is the opposite of intensity. Cell phones are to a workout what alcohol is to a drunk. Intensity means exerting your muscles and mind to full capacity on every rep of every set. There are three ways to jack up the intensity of your workout:

1. Lift heavier weights: By adding resistance and performing the same number of reps, you are forcing your muscles to work harder. For cardio, that means raising the incline and speed on the treadmill and the resistance on a stationary bike.
2. Lift the same weights for more reps: If you do 80 lbs for 10 reps, doing 80 lbs for 12 reps will strengthen the muscle. In the case of a cardio workout, run the same speed for a longer distance.
3. Train faster with less rest in between sets: Combine two, three, or even four exercises back-to-back-to-back-to-back and finish your workout faster and with better results.

Unless you're a competitive powerlifter, there is no reason to ever do just one set of an exercise and then rest. You should be doing supersets for the entire workout, which is two exercises performed back to back with no rest in between. The quality of a workout depends on intensity, and nothing destroys intensity faster than the constant start and stop from straight sets. Supersets keep you moving from one task to the next and prevent you from looking at your phone. Once you lose focus on the workout and start texting, the intensity is gone and you have to start back up from zero. Supersets, tri-sets, and giant sets all prevent this from happening. If equipment is limited, it doesn't matter. It's easy to superset lateral raises with crunches or hammer curls with leg raises. Abdominal exercises can always be superset with other exercises, and we could all use more work on our abs. At the minimum, you should complete 15 total sets in a 30-minute period and 30 sets in an hour.

## THE MAGIC NUMBER OF REPS

"Low reps for size, high reps for cuts. Low reps for size, high reps for cuts!" I've been hearing this since the late-'80s, when men had mullets and wore muscle tanks and women brandished perms and donned leotards. While their fashion sense was superior, their training advice was as bad then as it is today. Sadly, muscles do not magically grow from moving a bar two to four times, nor do they get shredded, sliced, or diced by reaching the number fifteen. To have "cuts"—also known as muscular definition—your body fat must be low, or your "cuts" will be concealed in blubber.

At the molecular level, low reps (1–5) stimulate myofibrillar hypertrophy, an increase in size and number of myosin filament in the muscle tissue. This style of training leads to increases in strength but does not build much muscle mass as effectively as moderate reps in the 6–12 range might do. Moderate reps cause sarcoplasmic hypertrophy, which means an increase in sarcoplasm in the muscle. And what is sarcoplasm, Andrew? Sarcoplasm is the cytoplasm of striated muscle cells; cytoplasm, if you recall 9th-grade biology, is all of the material in a cell minus the nucleus. Sarcoplasmic growth is the reason that bodybuilders look so big, even though it doesn't necessarily translate into strength. Yes, sometimes they are all show and no go. High reps in the 15–20 range empty the muscle's glycogen stores, which is the carbohydrates stored in the muscle. Though this sounds unfortunate, a muscle depleted in glycogen is forced to increase future glycogen stores, which leads to muscle growth and the release of anabolic hormones.

Since high reps, low reps, and moderate reps all have their advantages, which one should people use to maximize results? The answer is moderate reps and high reps, and the key is mixing up workouts so that one features reps in the 6–12 rep range and then the following workout stays in the 15–20 range. "But when do I get to max out on bench press?" You don't. You're not 18 anymore, and super-low reps with maximum weight increases your risk of injury exponentially. And if your ego is so frail that you must max out on your bench press to sleep at night, I know a wonderful therapist who takes insurance.

## COMPOUND EXERCISES WORK BEST

If you are searching for the best exercises to lose weight and build muscle, don't look any further than compound exercises. These are the ones that require the most energy to perform because they utilize several different muscle groups at once. Squats, lunges, deadlifts, pull-ups, clean and presses, bench presses, dips, and bent-over rows burn the most calories and will bring the most substantial results because they engage the greatest amount of muscle fiber. No matter what your level of fitness, these are the exercises around which your workout routine should always be based. They should also be performed first in your workout, long before any isolation movements are done.

When you perform a squat, you are forced to contract every muscle group, whereas the leg press machine limits tension to only your legs. You can wave to someone and carry on a conversation while on the leg press, but try that while squatting, and you will need a team of paramedics to peel you off the gym floor. For the same reason, the pulldown is inferior to a pull-up because you don't have to expend as much energy to pull your bodyweight through space. Of course, many people can't pull themselves up, and therein lies the beauty of the pulldown. If you have injuries that prohibit you from doing compound movements such as squats, that is one thing; but if you are just lazy and don't want to endure the heavy breathing and exertion that these movements require, you will never reach your full physical potential.

## THE PUMP

When you lift weights, blood rushes to the muscles to deliver oxygen and remove lactic acid so that the muscles can continue to contract. This is known as "the pump," and the muscles become much larger than they are when at rest. In *Pumping Iron,* Arnold Schwarzenegger compared the feeling of "the pump" to an orgasm. He said, "It's like having sex with a 'vuhmen' and 'coming.'" I disagree with Arnold and believe that the "pump" is more comparable to foreplay because during both the pump and foreplay, various parts of the body become engorged with blood, expand in size, and harden. Since the orgasm is the sudden discharge of sexual tension causing the added size to subside, it is unlike the pump, which causes the muscle to remain full of blood and fortify long after the workout.

The pump is a great way to gauge the quality of your workout, and if your muscles are flat and not expanding, you are either not isolating the muscle properly, you are dehydrated, and/or you do not have enough carbohydrates in your muscles. This is one of the reasons that it is so important to stay hydrated throughout the workout and eat a low glycemic complex carbohydrate at least an hour before heading to the gym. Specifically, oatmeal, brown rice, and sweet potatoes are fantastic for getting a pump and sustaining energy for the duration of the workout. To maximize the pump, I highly recommend drop sets on the last set of an exercise—when you can no longer do one more repetition with a given weight, lighten the weight just enough so that you can keep pumping out reps. When the muscles fails, lighten the weight even more and keep going. When your muscles are pumped with blood and appear much larger than normal, think of it as a preview of your future physique.

**MUSCLE SORENESS**

When John Cougar Mellencamp first performed the hit song "Hurt So Good," bodybuilders all over the world swore he was referring to the soreness one feels after an intense leg workout. Later, they would be disappointed to learn that the song was actually about a girl that he fell in love with. Never mind that! Soreness after a workout is healthy and means that you stimulated a muscle with the right amount of intensity. The soreness usually takes place 12–48 hours after the workout and is the most severe when you first begin a workout routine. Also known as DOMS (delayed onset muscle soreness), the pain typically last 2–5 days and is the result of small tears in the muscle from excessive stretching known as microtrauma.[1] This is a very different soreness than the one you experience during a workout when lactic acid builds up in the muscle at the end of a set. Unlike the 30–45-second rest period that the latter calls for, one must wait a few days for the tears in the muscle to heal and recover before training that muscle again. If you rush to train an already sore muscle, you will be much weaker and significantly raise your chances of injury.

It is possible to train too intensely, which I have made the mistake of doing several times in my life, and usually on leg day. Intense, high-volume leg workouts have left me sore and limping for up to two weeks! I was clearly overtraining and learned to cut back on the volume or risk a relapse in soreness and horror. At the same time, I have undertrained a muscle and it does not get sore because it was not stimulated enough. "No pain, no gain" really rings true. The longer you have been training, the harder it is to stimulate muscle growth and requires constantly changing your workout.

## WEIGHTS BEFORE CARDIO

People often question whether you should do cardio before weights, weights before cardio, cardio and weights together, or just stay home and screw it. The answer: weights before cardio. Why? Because if you do cardio first, your muscles will be fatigued by the time you hit the weights, and you won't be able to lift as much and your form will suffer. A recent study in the Journal of Strength and Conditioning Research tested three different workout styles against one another. One workout was strength training alone, another was strength training after cycling, and the third was strength training after running. Not surprisingly, they observed that the exercisers did fewer reps with the same poundage when they lifted weights after running and cycling.[2]

Another reason to lift first is that weight training uses the glycogen in your muscles as its energy source to pump blood into the muscle. By the end of the weight routine, your muscles have fewer carbohydrates to utilize before switching over to fat as its primary energy source. Since cardio is designed to keep your heart healthy and burn fat, it makes sense to burn fat from the very beginning. If your goal is to lose weight and build lean muscle, a perfect workout would be 30 minutes of weights followed by 30 minutes of cardio.

## MINDLESS MULTITASKING

When time is your adversary and your boss is an imbecile, you may be yelled at for not getting enough done at work and even hear, "You need to learn how to multitask." Nothing could be further from the truth, as studies have shown multitasking to reduce performance, increase anxiety, and possibly cause brain damage. Researchers at the University of Sussex in the UK compared the amount of time people spend on multiple devices, such as on a cell phone texting while also watching TV, and found that high multitaskers had less brain density in the anterior cingulate cortex, a region responsible for empathy as well as cognitive and emotional control.[3]

Multitasking has become commonplace in the gym as trainers instruct their clients to lunge, then curl, and then press for one big, strange repetition. The time that they save by combining exercises fails to make up for the loss in efficiency. Instead of doing one exercise with maximum focus, the client attempts to juggle three like an untrained clown. Pick one! Lunge, curl, or press. I've even seen people combine the leg press machine with incline dumbbell presses. It's a train wreck to witness and an injury waiting to happen.

## TOO SICK TO TRAIN?

"Should I work out if I'm sick?" Though the answer is an unequivocal "no," I can't say that I always abide by that rule. To me, when a doctor says that I should take a week off from training, I always seem to hear, "Get back in the gym and train!" Stubborn as a mule, I'm proof that brains and brawn don't go together. If you are sick with a cold, your immune system is fighting a virus and the idea of "sweating it out" is nonsense. Exercise will stress your body further, and it will take longer to recover and get healthy. Other criteria to consider include the following:

Are you contagious? If you are sneezing, coughing, or wheezing, you will make everyone around you sick. All you have to do is cough into your hands and grab a weight, and you have successfully spread the epidemic. Unless you are working out in your own private space, stay away from the gym.

How long and hard will you work out? If you are sick and must work out, be prepared to take it easy and listen to your body. If you are somebody who must go all out and push their body to the extreme, stay home and rest. Soon enough, you will back in the gym at full speed and you won't make everyone around you sick.

## MY TEN COMMANDMENTS FOR TRAINING

1. Always maintain perfect form and never sacrifice it for heavy weight.
2. Train weak points more often than strong points and earlier in the workout when you're fresh.
3. Train for 45 minutes to an hour. Once an hour is reached, turn around and go home.
4. Constantly change up your workout every 6 to 8 weeks and keep your body guessing.
5. Always pick free weights over machines.
6. Lift weights before doing cardio.
7. Always warm up a muscle properly before using heavy weights.
8. Take one second to complete the positive part of the movement and spend two seconds on the negative.
9. Take at least one day off a week to rest and recuperate.
10. Complete 30 sets in one hour, 15 sets in half an hour.

# CHAPTER 10
# Building the Classic Physique

## PROPORTION

The goal of weight training is to build and define all of the muscle groups so that they are in perfect proportion and nothing stands out. Historically, the Grecian ideal says that the arms, calves, and neck should all be the same size, the neck should be half the size of the waist, and the thighs half the size of the chest. Has anyone ever achieved these perfect proportions? Yes, but he

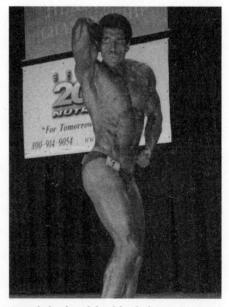

*Ripped, sliced, and diced for the beauty pageant.*

stands still in Florence and is made of marble.

## TRAINING ROUTINES

Long before steroids and CrossFit, bodybuilders and strongmen performed full body workouts three times a week to build muscular size and strength. Then along came the split routine where the body was broken in half and trained over two separate workouts, one for the upper and one for the lower body. With this workout plan, the lifters trained four days a week in order to hit each muscle group twice. Still unsatisfied, bodybuilders such as Arnold Schwarzenegger and Lou Ferrigno sliced the cake yet again and added a third workout to cover the entire body, hitting each muscle twice a week and now training six days. This workout style remained popular for a while until today's generation decided to cut down their workload even further and reduce output to one muscle group per day. If history is any indicator of the future, soon we will be training each muscle group once every two weeks, followed by monthly and, God help us, annually. I don't even want to imagine what the steroid cycles will look like by then, but I am fairly certain that funeral parlors will double their workload and be open seven days to accommodate the high demand.

To compare workout styles and determine a winner is to compare children and pick a favorite. Each has their own strengths and weaknesses, and certain body types will respond differently to each type of training. Much like diet, there is no way to know right off the bat which workout will be most effective for you. The only way to find out is to try different routines. You are the lab, experiment, and scientist all rolled up into one, and it is up to you (and your trainer, if you have one) to figure out what your body responds to best. In this chapter, I will include many different workout routines with which you can experiment. I have used all of these routines for years and have seen my clients benefit from them, as well.

When you look at the top physiques of the past 100 years, you'll quickly notice that the most massive and muscular bodybuilders are the ones today that mainly adhere to a split routine in which they train one to two muscle groups daily. Since drug use is so much more prevalent and advanced than it was 50 years ago, one can presume that the chemicals have played a much larger role in the development than the workouts. After all, bodybuilders perform the same exercises from fifty years ago, but the vials and syringes carry something much more potent.

## THE BEGINNER ROUTINE

When you first begin weight training, you will make rapid gains in strength and muscle tone, since the resistance is new to the body. For the first three months of training, I recommend three full-body workouts per week with a day rest in between each workout. On the off days from weights, do 20-30 minutes of cardio. One day per week, take a full day off from weights and cardio. For each workout, you will perform one exercise per body part for three sets each, and the routine should take approximately 45 minutes to complete. On each exercise, increase the weight for each set while dropping down the number of repetitions. Below you'll find a sample full-body workout.

### Monday

Incline Dumbbell Press: 3 sets of 12, 10, 8

Lat Pulldowns: 3 sets of 15, 12, 10

Squats: 3 sets of 15, 12, 10

Lateral Raises: 3 sets of 15, 12, 10

Barbell Curls: 3 sets of 12, 10, 8

Tricep Cable Pushdowns: 3 sets of 15, 12, 10

Crunches: 3 sets of 20

**Wednesday**

Bench Press: 3 sets of 12, 10, 8

Cable Rows: 3 sets of 15, 12, 10

Pullovers: 3 sets of 15, 12, 10

Barbell Upright Rows: 3 sets of 12, 10, 8

Incline Dumbbell Curls: 3 sets of 12, 10, 8

Lying Triceps Extensions: 3 sets of 12, 10, 8

Leg Press: 3 sets of 20, 15, 15

Incline Crunches: 3 sets of 20

Leg Raises: 3 sets of 20

**Friday**

Flat Dumbbell Flyes: 3 sets of 12, 10, 8

One-Arm Dumbbell Rows: 3 sets of 12, 10, 8

Rear Lateral Raises: 3 sets of 12

Hammer Curls: 3 sets of 12, 10, 8

Dumbbell Kickbacks: 3 sets of 12, 10, 8

Reverse Curls: 3 sets of 15, 12, 10

Lunges: 4 sets of 12, 10, 8, 8 reps

Leg Raises: 3 sets of 25

**ACTIVE REST**

In between sets, you should rest 30 to 45 seconds, but use that time to stretch the muscle being worked. For example, after each set of a chest exercise, do a doorway stretch, where you place your arm on a wall at shoulder height and turn away from the wall, straightening your arm to a full stretch. Hold each stretch for 20 seconds.

For shoulders, reach your right arm across your body and hold it straight. With your left arm, grab your right elbow and pull it across your body toward your chest.

For your back, lean over, reach out, and grab a vertical column or rail and pull it as hard as you can, stretching all of your back muscles.

For your quadriceps, stand up on your right foot, grab your left foot with your left hand, and pull it up behind you so that your heel touches your butt.

For hamstrings, stand with the leg to be stretched just in front of the other one. Bend the back knee and lean forward from the hips. Place your hands on the bent leg's thigh, to balance yourself. If you can't feel a stretch, lean farther forward and tilt your pelvis forward.

Biceps: Stand with your hands clasped behind your back. Turn your clasped palms downward, then lift your hands up until you feel tension in your biceps.

Triceps: Reach your right hand behind your head with your elbow pointed up over your head. Grasp your elbow with your left hand and gently pull.

## THE INTERMEDIATE ROUTINE

After three months of abiding by the beginner routine, it's time to add a fourth workout each week and split up the workouts so that you train the entire body over two workouts instead of one. You will do two exercises per muscle group and superset the workout so that you do two exercises back-to-back with no rest. After each superset, rest for 30-45 seconds until you catch your breath. Increase weight on each successive set of an exercise. You will follow a two days on/one day off, two days on/ two days off schedule, with three cardio sessions to go along with the weight workouts.

### Day 1: Chest, Back, Legs
Flat Chest Press: 4 sets of 15, 12, 10, 8

Superset with Lat Pulldowns: 4 sets of 15, 12, 10, 10

Incline Dumbbell Flyes: 3 sets of 12, 10, 8

Superset with Cable Rows: 3 sets of 12, 10, 8

Pullovers: 3 sets of 15

Superset with Squats: 4 sets of 20, 15, 12, 10

Crunches: 4 sets of 20

### Day 2: Shoulders, Biceps, Triceps, Abs
Seated Overhead Dumbbell Press: 4 sets of 12, 10, 8, 8

Superset with Dumbbell Lateral Raises: 4 sets 12, 10, 8, 8

Hammer Curls: 3 sets of 12

Superset with Triceps Cable Pushdowns: 4 sets of 15, 12, 10, 8

Incline Curls: 3 sets of 12, 10, 8

Superset with Skull Crushers: 3 sets of 10

Leg raises: 3 sets of 20

### Day 3: Cardio
Options: 30 minutes of treadmill, bike, StepMill, or StairMaster

### Day 4: Chest, Back, Legs
Incline Barbell Press: 4 sets of 15, 12, 10, 8

Superset with Wide Grip Pull-Ups: 4 sets: do as many as you can (use assisted pull-up machine if necessary)

Flat Dumbbell Press: 3 sets of 12, 10, 8

Superset with Bent Rows: 3 sets of 15, 12, 10

Leg Press: 4 sets of 20, 15, 10, 8

Stiff-Legged Deadlifts: 3 sets of 12, 10, 8

Crunches: 4 sets of 25 reps

### Day 5: Shoulders, Biceps, Triceps, Abs

Upright Rows: 3 sets of 12, 10, 8

Superset with Dumbbell Lateral Raises: 3 sets of 12, 10, 8

Barbell Curls: 3 sets of 12, 10, 8

Superset with Dips: 3 sets of 15 reps

Incline Dumbbell Curls: 3 sets of 10, 8, 6

Superset with Rope Triceps Extensions (Facing away from Pulley): 3 sets of 12, 10, 8

Incline Leg Raises: 4 sets of 20

Hyperextensions: 3 sets of 15

### Day 6: Cardio

Options: 30 minutes of treadmill, bike, StepMill, or StairMaster

### Day 7: Rest

## THE ONE-MUSCLE-PER-DAY ROUTINE

If you have the luxury of working out five or six days a week and want to make improvements, I'd suggest a one-muscle-per-day training split. By training only one muscle per workout, you can really attack it with full focus and maximum intensity. I learned this style of training from pro bodybuilder Ali Malla, who trained me when I was 19 years old. When you look at the workout split below, you will notice that I devote an entire day to just "Abs." This is because they are so often neglected and thrown in at the end of a workout as a footnote, and I prefer to prioritize the abs and give them their own day. Each muscle group will take between 30 and 40 minutes to train thoroughly. This makes it easy to fit each workout into a schedule and also allows time for cardio, which I recommend doing three days a week for at least 30 minutes.

Here is the workout split that I use:

**Monday:** Shoulders

**Tuesday:** Arms

**Wednesday:** Legs

**Thursday:** Chest

**Friday:** Back

**Saturday:** Abs

**Sunday:** Rest

[Note: I pick four exercises per muscle group for 3–4 sets each and always vary the workout.]

## SUPERHERO SHOULDERS

Long before Marvel Comics, there was Baccio Bandinelli and Michelangelo. The sculptors of "Hercules" and "David," respectively, they stressed certain muscles in their quest for the perfect male form. The main focus was on shoulders, abs, and calves. The wider the shoulders, the smaller the waist appeared. The side deltoid is the muscle that creates this illusion.

This beautiful slab of tissue makes women look incredible in a strapless dress and makes men fill out a suit.

If you want to look like a superhero, you must develop your X Factor. Andrew, what the hell are you talking about? Okay, if you draw a line from each shoulder to the opposite foot, you have an X. The wider the X, the more you resemble Superman, got it? Here are two shoulder workouts to alternate that will enhance your X Factor:

**Workout #1**
Dumbbell Lateral Raises: 4 sets of 12, 10, 8, 6 reps (2 drop sets on last set of exercise)
Upright Rows (Shoulder-Width Grip): 3 sets of 12, 10, 8 reps
Seated Dumbbell Press: 3 sets of 10, 8, 6 reps
Rear Lateral Raises: 3 sets of 12, 10, 8 reps (1 drop set)

**Workout #2**
Standing Barbell Press: 4 sets of 15, 12, 10, 8 reps
Seated Dumbbell Laterals: 3 sets of 12, 10, 8 reps
Dumbbell Front Raises: 3 sets of 12, 10, 8 reps
Dumbbell Upright Rows: 3 sets of 12, 10, 8 reps

## THE GUN SHOW

A pair of sculpted arms look good on a beach, in a t-shirt, or etched in stone. When somebody says, "Make a muscle," we instantly flex our bicep. Because of this reflex, many people train their biceps into oblivion and neglect their triceps, which make up ⅔ of the arm. When a woman is told that she has "grandma arms," the asshole is referring to the flab that covers her triceps. To make the biceps and triceps look their best, I recommend

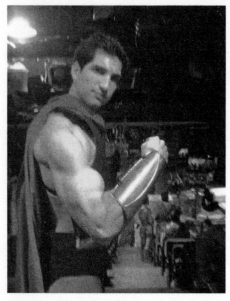

*Flexing as a Spartan on* SNL.

that you superset both muscles, meaning a set of biceps followed by a set of triceps. By pumping up your biceps, your triceps will work harder and more efficiently due to the cushioning effect of the muscles. The goal is to get as much blood in the upper arm as possible and then go home to feed and then rest the damaged muscle tissue. It then grows back bigger and stronger, and people tell you how ripped your arms look. Here are the workouts to build balanced, sculpted arms:

**Workout #1**

Incline Dumbbell Curls: 4 sets of 12, 10, 8, 6 reps (add weight each set)

Triceps Cable Pushdowns: 15, 12, 10, 8 reps (2 drop sets on last set)

Hammer curls: 3 sets of 10, 8, 8 reps

Skull Crushers: 3 sets of 10, 8, 6 reps

Standing Concentration Curls: 3 sets of 8 reps

Overhead Dumbbell Extensions: 4 sets of 12, 10, 10, 8 reps

**Workout #2**

EZ Bar Curls: 4 sets of 12, 10, 8, 6 reps

Cable Triceps Extensions (Facing away from Pulley): 4 sets of 12, 10, 8, 8 reps

Seated Alternating Dumbbell Curls: 3 sets of 12, 10, 8 reps

Close-Grip Bench Press: 3 sets of 12, 10, 8 reps

Cable Rope Curls: 3 sets of 15 reps

Dumbbell Kickbacks: 3 sets of 12, 10, 8 reps

## THE CEPHALIC VEIN WORKOUT

Recently, a male client of mine told me that he wanted "that vein." I asked "What vein?" He said, "You know, that vein," and pointed to my right bicep. I quickly realized he was talking about the vein that runs from your deltoid down through your bicep and into your forearm. It is called the cephalic vein and makes your arms look really good in t-shirts. For muscles to appear vascular, your body fat has to be low or the muscle will be concealed under the fat. If you are lean, mean, and vain, and want vascular biceps, here is the workout for you:

Hammer Curls: 4 sets of 12, 10, 8, 8 reps

Reverse Curls: 4 sets of 15 reps

Reverse Preacher Curls: 3 sets of 15, 12, 10 reps

[Note: Take 30 seconds in between sets for each of the exercises noted above.]

## THE LIVE FROM HELL LEG WORKOUT

There are no muscles more painful to train than those of the legs, which explains why so many people have great upper bodies and puny lower ones. While training chest and arms can be exhilarating, leg day will test your character and will to live. The deep burning pain in the quadriceps at the very end of a set of lunges or squats has to be second only to childbirth, on which, of course, I cannot comment. That said, the benefits of leg training are vast. There is no better way to burn body fat than by training your legs with heavy weights. Here is a leg workout that you will feel for days.

Leg Extensions: 3 sets of 20 reps (very light warmup sets)

Squats: 4 sets of 20, 15, 12, 10 reps (add weight each set)

Stiff-Legged Deadlifts: 3 sets of 12, 10, 8

Hack Squats: 3 sets of 15

Dumbbell Lunges: 4 sets of 12

Standing Calf Raises: 4 sets of 20

Seated Calf Raises: 3 sets of 25

## TWO CHESTNUTS

A wise man once told me, "Any woman can have big boobs, but a woman with a nice ass takes care of herself." I've always agreed with that statement because a nice ass requires a woman to eat right, exercise, or be born in Brazil. Here is a workout for anyone who wants a nice butt that resembles two chestnuts:

Wide Stance Leg Press: 3 sets of 20 reps

Squats: 4 sets of 15 reps

Dumbbell Lunges: 4 sets of 15 reps

Stiff-Legged Deadlifts: 4 sets of 15 reps

## TEN SETS OF TEN

The most widely held excuse for not working out is lack of time, which has led to "quickies" known as "The 7-Minute

Workout" and even a "2-Minute Workout." Two minutes? It takes me longer than that just to untangle my headphones. If time is your nemesis, I suggest getting your ass in the gym and doing 10 sets of 10 reps of squats. That's it! It shouldn't take more than 20 minutes, and it's the best workout you can get in that time period. I do this once every couple of weeks and have experienced great results from "the king of all exercises."

Find a weight that is challenging for 10 reps of squats and do 10 sets of deep, in the bucket, ass to heel squats. Check that—just go low enough so that your upper thighs are parallel to the ground (I just wanted to say ass to heel). I don't care if you do your squats with free weights, the Smith Machine, or against the wall with a stability ball, just do them! Take no more than 45 seconds of rest in between sets and remember to keep your shoulders back, chest up, and breathe!

Ten sets of ten, go!


## TREASURE CHEST

Like Times Square, the bench press remains the crossroads to the gym world. The overtly cliché exercise provides bragging rights to meatheaded shitstacks around the world who petition one another, "Yo man, how much can you bench?" Based on the gorilla's inflated response, his value as an alpha male is defined.

Not only do I think the bench press is overrated, I don't even think it's the most effective chest exercise. I have always found the incline press and dips to be more rewarding. Now, don't get me wrong, the bench press has its place in lifting, but it's not the "end-all, be-all" king of exercises.

Male or female, here are two chest workouts that will help your development significantly:

## Workout #1

Barbell Incline Presses: 4 sets of 15, 12, 10, 8 reps

Incline Dumbbell Flyes: 4 sets of 12, 10, 8, 6 reps

Dumbbell Flat Presses: 3 sets of 12, 10, 8

Dumbbell Pullovers: 3 sets of 15 reps

*Add weight on each successive set

## Workout #2

Flat Bench Press: 4 sets of 15, 10, 8, 6 reps

Incline Dumbbell Press: 4 sets of 12, 10, 8, 6 reps

Fly Dumbbell Flyes: 3 sets of 12, 10, 8 reps

Cable Crossovers: 4 sets of 15, 12, 10, 8 reps

*Add weight on each successive set.

## THE V SHAPE

After the legs, the back muscles are the second largest and the second most neglected muscles of the body. Since you can't see your back when you look into a mirror, it is not a priority to the average trainee. Unfortunately, by ignoring your back and giving ultimate attention to your chest, you develop an imbalance that not only looks bad but will negatively affect your health. If the majority of mass is on your chest, you will be "front-heavy," which will destroy your posture and likely cause lower back pain. This is the reason that many women with extremely large chests choose to get a breast reduction. Train your back as often and as intensely as the rest of your muscles. Here are the workouts to build your lats and "V torso":

## Workout #1

Deadlifts: 4 sets of 15, 12, 10, 8 reps

Wide Grip Lat Pulldowns: 4 sets of 15, 12, 10, 8 reps

Cable Rows: 3 sets of 12, 10, 8 reps

One-Arm Dumbbell Rows: 3 sets of 12, 10, 8 reps

Hyperextensions: 3 sets of 15 reps

*Add weight on each successive set.

**Workout #2**

Pull-ups: 3 sets each of wide grip, reverse grip, and triangle grip (as many reps as possible)

Barbell Bent Rows: 4 sets of 15, 12, 10, 8 reps

Pullovers: 3 sets of 15 reps

## PULL-UPS OR PROZAC?

When I'm feeling depressed and the interior of my oven appears a welcome environment, I force myself to go to the gym and do pull-ups. Besides being an incredible exercise for your back, biceps, and shoulders, the motion itself acts as an antidepressant. Physically, you're lifting your body up, and mentally, your mood follows. You get "high" in a number of ways and leave the gym in euphoric delight.

I recommend 3 sets of 10, using three different grips—wide grip, close grip, and reverse grip—for a total of 9 sets.

[Note: If you are a weakling and can't do pull-ups, use one of those assisted pull-up machines. Remember to always pull with the elbows on all back exercises and to crunch your shoulder blades together at the top.]

## THE EIGHT-PACK WORKOUT

Everyone wants a six pack, the six bricks that solidify an ego. Don't be like everyone else, though. Go for an eight pack! That way, if you fall short, you'll still have at least six. That also means you need to do giant sets. Yes, giant sets! Lawrence Taylor created them, and they're four exercises performed back-to-back, nonstop, with no rest. Once (if) you get through the fourth exercise, take a minute rest and question your existence. If you can handle the pain, here's my eight-pack ab routine. Do a total of three giant sets (four exercises back-to-back equals one giant set), and within a month, male or female, you'll wear nothing but cutoff shirts. Enough talk, here's what you do:

1. Leg Raises
2. Knee-ins
3. Crunches
4. Bar Twists

**Leg Raises:** Lie on a flat bench with your butt placed at the bottom edge. Keeping your legs straight, feet together, and your lower back on the bench, raise your legs straight up until they're perpendicular to your body. Then lower your legs below the level of the bench. Exhale as the legs come up, inhale as they go down. Do 3 sets of 25 reps.

**Knee-ins:** Sitting upright at the end of a bench, grab the bench at your sides, and pull your knees into your body and your upper body into your knees. Think of it as an accordion and blow all the air out when the knees come in. Do 3 sets of 25 reps.

**Crunches:** Lying on the floor, preferably a mat, put your legs up on a bench. Now, place your hands behind your head or fingers behind your ears (more difficult) and crunch straight up toward the ceiling. Big exhale at the top and then come down slowly without letting your head touch the ground. Do 3 sets of 25 reps.

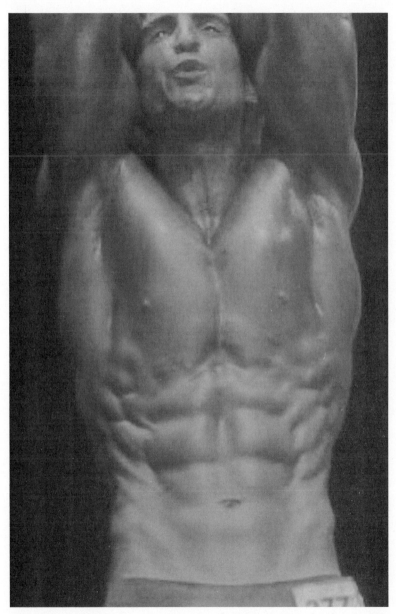

*Eight is better than six.*

**Bar Twists:** Sit at the edge of a bench, holding a bar or broomstick behind your head. Now twist back and forth, looking behind you on each rep as you flex the obliques. As you get more comfortable, increase your speed. This exercise is the "love handles'" worst enemy. Remember to exhale on each rep. Do 3 sets of 50 reps.

This routine should be performed 3 days a week on an empty stomach.

## THE PHIL HERNON ROUTINE

Phil Hernon, a legendary pro bodybuilder and mentor whom I mentioned earlier in the book, adheres to a full body workout style in which he trains the entire body each session and picks one exercise per body part for one set every single day. If you do it right, you will not need a rest day because you will not be doing the kind of volume that requires taking time off. As easy as one set per body part may sound, Phil takes each set to failure, and the workout is nonstop with very little rest. The beauty of this routine is that it can be done for the rest of your life and allows for creativity. The exercises are compound movements done with free weights and vary from day to day like the repetitions. Some days it is heavy weights with lower reps (8–10) and other days it is lighter weights with high reps (15–20). He keeps his body guessing and has one of the best physiques in the history of bodybuilding.

## TRAIN IN OPPOSITION

To keep your workouts stimulating to both your mind and your body, it is imperative to constantly switch up the routines and pair different muscles and exercises together. One of the best ways to do this is to train in opposition. By that, I mean training opposing muscle groups together such as chest with back, biceps with triceps, quads with hamstrings, and abs with lower back. By pumping more blood into the chest, it makes the back stronger because it provides a "cushioning effect" in that upper body region. The more blood in the muscle, the more oxygen to the muscle, and the stronger the muscle!

Here's how you do this:

Do a set of chest, followed immediately by a set of back, and then rest a minute. Do three supersets for 15 reps, and you'll get an amazing pump.

Here are my favorite exercise combos:

Chest and Back: Dumbbell Incline Chest Press/Lat Pulldowns

Biceps and Triceps: Dumbbell Incline Curls/Lying Triceps Extension

Quads and Hamstrings: Stiff-Legged Deadlifts/Lunges

Shoulders: Front Delts with Side Delts; Dumbbell Overhead Press/Lateral Raises

Abs with Lower Back: Leg Raises/Hyperextensions

## WHEN TRAINING GOES OFF THE RAILS

If you don't train for balance and favor certain muscle groups, you will overdevelop those areas at the expense of other muscles, and your body will look like crap. Here are some of the most common unbalanced body types you see at the gym:

**The No Neck:** This guy trains his traps far too often and overdevelops them, destroying any semblance of shoulder width. Go easy on the traps, hard on the side delts, and you will avoid this look.

**The Runner's Legs:** Since jogging focuses so heavily on the quadriceps, the hamstrings often lack development, which makes the legs look front-heavy. Make sure to balance this out with a steady diet of lying leg curls and stiff-legged deadlifts.

**The Bull Chest:** This guy bench presses and bench presses and bench presses some more. He walks around like a bull and suffers from Imaginary Lat Syndrome (ILS). His chest is huge, but his back is nonexistent. Similar to the quad-hamstring imbalance, this guy looks front-heavy and often has bad posture. Avoid this meatheaded shitstack look by training your back with equal intensity. Do pull-ups and rows along with your bench press.

**Mr. Chicken Legs:** If all you do is train upper body, you better never wear shorts. Instead, train your legs as often and with the same intensity as you train your upper body.

**The Block Waist:** This person has strong abdominals but overdeveloped obliques, which makes the waist wider. Avoid direct oblique work and focus on crunches and leg raises.

## DANGER ZONE

As a personal trainer, I often see other trainers allowing and sometimes instructing their clients to use the wrong form on certain exercises that can lead to serious injury. Like a guy driving against traffic with a beer in one hand and texting his girlfriend with the other, it is an accident waiting to happen and an easily avoidable one given the right guidance. With the personal training profession growing like wildfire, more and more actors are choosing to be a trainer over a waiter and thus keeping orthopedic surgeons gainfully employed. Here are the most common exercise mistakes that can lead a client out of the gym and onto an operating table:

1. **Lunges:** As the client lunges down, his knee is in front of his toe, putting added pressure on the ligaments. When you lunge, the front knee should always stay behind the toe.

2. **Deadlifts:** The client rounds her spine as she descends down with the weight and risks rupturing every disc in her lower back. Your lower back must always be arched.

3. **Lat Pulldown:** The client pulls the bar down to his stomach and works nothing but his biceps. The bar should be pulled to the top of your chest with your back slightly arched as you squeeze your shoulder blades together. On back exercises, always think "Pull with the elbows."

4. **Fast, loose form:** The client does biceps curls, swinging a heavy weight from point A to point B with her back bending and zero focus on the actual muscle. A bicep curl should be done with no swinging, perfect form, and taking two seconds on the negative part of the movement.

5. **Triceps Cable Pushdowns:** The elbows flare all over the place and the triceps receive very little, if any, stimulation. Elbows still, please.

6. **Squats:** The client has his back bent forward, taking the focus off of his ass and quads and onto the lower back. Shoulders back, chest up, and back straight.

7. **Running up and down the stairs:** Certain trainers make their clients run up and down a stairwell

with weights in their hands. Currently, a few of us trainers have a bet going over whose client will be the first to tumble down the long, narrow, uneven stairwell. Do step-ups on a bench and save yourself a lawsuit.

## INJURIES

Aging is a question of what doesn't hurt. You wake up every morning and do a systems check. Does my back hurt? No? Cool, I can stand up straight. Does my knee hurt? No? Good, I can walk. Unfortunately, as we get older, we do not get stronger. Our metabolism slows down, bones and muscles weaken, and our vital organs work harder and less efficiently. The goal is to strengthen the body and mind to maximize your fight against further injury. When you do get injured, it's just as important to learn to work around it as it is to let it heal. If you strain your shoulder, you can still train legs, abs, and perform cardio. If you hurt your lower back, you can still do certain exercises seated that will not exacerbate the injury. And if you hurt your knee, shoulder, and lower back, well, there are some really good movies streaming on Netflix that you should check out. The worst thing you can do is train through an injury, which will only make it worse. Listen to your body, which tells you everything you need to know.

If you do get injured and find that the muscle, tendon, or ligament is not healing on its own, go to a doctor and get it checked out. Do not go on WebMD and self-diagnose. Of course, that's what you're going to do, since we all hate going to the doctor and sitting in a waiting room for two hours. "Let's see here, I have a subcutaneous contusion." No idiot, you have a broken femur. When you suffer an injury, you can reduce swelling and promote healing by immediately adhering to RICE:

**Rest:** Take a break from any activity that will exacerbate the pain.

**Ice:** Apply an ice pack to the injury for 10–20 minutes at least three times a day for the first 48 hours. After that, apply heat to the area.

**Compression:** Wrap the injury (not too tight).

**Elevate:** Try to keep the injury elevated on a pillow above the level of your heart as often as possible.

Always stretch and warm up a muscle properly—if you are training your biceps, for example, don't come in from off the street and grab the 100-pound barbell and start curling away. Instead, grab the 40-pound bar and warm that muscle up. Let it stretch and contract and fill with blood. Then proceed to the 60-pound weight and do another set. Ease into the heavier weight; don't start with it.

## DYSFUNCTIONAL TRAINING

A style of training known as "Functional training" has taken over most gym chains as the vast majority of personal trainers employ this method, since it is what they are taught while obtaining their certification. What is functional training, you ask? The technical definition is training the body for activities performed in daily life. The actual definition should be any exercise that makes you look like a complete idiot, takes up too much space on the gym floor, and is a total waste of time. Popular "functional" exercises include one-legged squats, one-legged standing rows, and break dancer pushups. Yes, these are one-legged exercises because, obviously, we all stand on one leg in daily life. Or maybe functional training was just designed for those looking to improve in hopscotch? Whatever the case may be, functional trainers also love their colorful props and toys that include resistance bands, TRX, stability balls, slide boards, and battle ropes. To the untrained eye, these circus workouts may appear fun, innovative, and productive. However, anyone with a few years of training under his or her belt will realize that "functional training" is a dysfunctional mess.

Basic strength training is much more functional and a hundred times more effective than this sideshow that contaminates gyms around the globe. Why use one leg to squat when you were dealt two? You have that second leg for a reason, and I'm guessing it's to support half your body weight. Functional training also does not believe in training a muscle to failure, since in real life the muscles are seldom pushed to that point. That is precisely why you should train to failure! Why bother going to the gym at all if you are there to do exactly what you do at home? If you are looking to build a strong, aesthetic physique, do not waste your time with functional training. Trust me, doing push-ups on a stability ball or one-legged squats while standing on a balance board is neither fun nor effective. It's just dumb.

## WEAK POINT TRAINING

If you have chicken legs, hit the squat rack. Concave chest, hit the bench press. Under-developed brain, read a book (NOT this one). It is so important to focus on your weak points and train them FIRST. If you already have wide, sweeping lats, don't go overboard with the pull-ups. If you have ripped arms, there is no need to open the workout with barbell curls. Too many men strut around the gym with a big chest, huge arms, and no legs. Two chicken bones in motion is never an attractive site.

One should always strive for balance. Women, if you have perfect cleavage, don't sprint over to the pec-deck or cable crossover. You don't need more chest, but you may need more ass, so start squatting. A woman with a huge chest and no ass is the equivalent of a guy with massive arms and two chicken legs.

Weak point training can and should be applied to everyday life. My cooking used to be terrible, but with a few pointers and some high quality olive oil, it's now edible, even enjoyable. Similarly, my shoes seem to always land in the middle of the living room, but with my wife's guidance, they are kept by the front door. The sink no longer overflows with dishes since she taught me to place them immediately into the dishwasher. Work on your weak points, maintain your strong points, and everybody will benefit.

**Best Muscle-Building Exercises for Skinny People:**

Chest: Bench Press, Incline Dumbbell Press, Dips

Back: Wide Grip Pull-Ups, Bent over Rows, Deadlifts

Shoulders: Lateral Raises, Upright Rows

Biceps: Barbell Curls, Incline Dumbbell curls

Triceps: Lying Triceps Extension (Skull Crushers), Close-Grip Bench Press

Legs: Squats, Lunges, Stiff-Legged Deadlifts

## WEDDING DAY CRASH COURSE

For the past seven months since your engagement, you've celebrated with another one of your 500 girlfriends over dinner, drinks, and even more drinks. In other words, you've gained weight and have only eight weeks until judgment day.

Fear not, that is enough time to look amazing in your dress and make all of your single friends jealous. Here's how to do it:

1. Cut down on your bottle-of-wine-a-day drinking habit to only two nights a week and limit yourself to two drinks each night. Sounds awful, right? Not as awful as feeling fat on your wedding day.
2. Dinner should always be high in protein with a leafy green vegetable nearby.
3. Cut all breads, pasta, and anything else that tastes good until your honeymoon.
4. Perform cardio four days a week for a minimum of 30 minutes. Stepmill, treadmill, or a spinning class works best.
5. Don't be a Bridezilla! Stress releases the hormone cortisol, which makes you stuff your face with donuts.
6. Drink at least half a gallon of water a day.
7. Do lunges! Lots and lots of lunges. Lunges are to an ass what Monet is to a canvas.
8. Do a full-body weight routine three days a week, with an emphasis on the shoulders, arms, and legs.
9. Have a lot of premarital sex with your fiancé. Sex burns calories and will relax you so that you make clear choices on which centerpiece goes best with the mauve tablecloths.
10. Do legs raises and crunches daily. A small waist will accentuate your round shoulders and make you look even more beautiful.

## CARDIO

Some people do their cardio in a classroom setting, while others prefer it in isolation. To me, there are few things more miserable than doing cardio. Spending thirty minutes on a sliding rubber floor or pedaling endlessly on a bike that doesn't move doesn't excite me. The same goes for the moving staircase and the rowing machine. I prefer to lift weights for cardio in a non-stop fashion that really gets my heart rate up. The important thing is doing some form of cardio at least three days a week for a minimum of twenty minutes. Yes, it will help you burn calories, but you are doing it for your heart health. Never forget that! Luckily, there are numerous ways to do your cardio and even some that do not involve a machine. Among them:

Walking: When people ask me what my favorite thing to do in New York City is, I always say "taking a walk." You will see and hear more interesting things in a two-block radius in New York City than you would if you walked through all of Long Island. I keep a brisk pace and walk for 45 minutes. If the weather does not permit me to walk outside, I'll suffer on a treadmill and walk at a 4.0 pace on a 5.0 grade incline. Walking can burn 400 calories in an hour.

Jumping Rope: Channel your inner Rocky Balboa and jump rope for 30 minutes. Jumping rope is a massive calorie burner and more stimulating than the treadmill.

Sprinting: By sprinting for 30 seconds or a minute followed by walking for 30 seconds, you can make cardio less monotonous and burn a ton of calories. If you sprint 100 yards 10 times, you can burn up to 500 calories.

## Cardio Classes

Like most women, my wife prefers workout classes over exercising alone. Maybe it's the structure, the music, or having someone tell her exactly what to do. Maybe it's the energy and competition of the other women. All I know is that workout classes fill up fast in New York City, and like a typical male, I just don't get it. My wife does something called "ClassPass," which offers a wide variety of classes ranging from yoga to pole dancing. You pay a monthly fee and then mix and match classes as you see fit. If you prefer classes and bore easily, I highly recommend ClassPass. When you sign up online for a class, you will be charged if you cancel the day of, so the motivation to exercise is stronger. The music the instructor plays is just as important, if not more so, than the exercises themselves. If Beyonce, Eminem, and Jay-Z are on the playlist, my wife will enjoy the spin class and most likely go back, while country music will send her fleeing for the exit. If you're wondering why women prefer workout classes more than men do, I could speculate that it's because women take instruction better and are far less competitive when it comes to exercise. Women also tend to enjoy being in a group setting more than most men do. When my wife travels or goes out to dinner with her friends, it is not uncommon for the reservation to be for for eight or nine people. I don't think I've had dinner with more than three other guys since I was a freshman in college. Many of us are loners and prefer being home alone watching sports. Okay, maybe that's just me? This may also be why more women than men use personal trainers. The "typical guy" who won't ask for directions when he's lost is the same guy who does every exercise wrong in the gym. He'd rather heave a heavy weight around with terrible form than dare ask another person how to do it properly.

## The Elliptical

The elliptical machine is the American dream of fitness, as it allows one to catch up on reality TV and exert minimal effort while still under the guise of exercise. Lauded by many for its "joint-friendly" design, dozens of gym zombies glide endlessly along on the elliptical as they shift their focus back and forth between Snapchat, Tinder, and *The Real Housewives of Orange County.* Each zombie resembles the next with the same blank stare and fixed cyclical gliding motion as Big Brother looks down on the Orwellian machine.

If you are under eighty, have a fully functioning meniscus, and have not drunk a quart of vodka prior to working out, there is no reason to ever use this martian device. Instead, hop on a treadmill, set the speed at 3.5 with an incline of 8.0, and walk briskly for 30 minutes. If you don't like treadmills, ride the stationary bike. If the stationary bike doesn't interest you, use the rowing machine. If you're walking on an incline on the treadmill, squeeze your ass hard on each stride. When spinning, flex your quads and hamstrings. Don't go through the motions. Put your mind into it!

When it comes to cardio, some machines are better than others, and a few are just a complete waste of time. Here are my Top Ten Cardio Machines, from most effective to the biggest piece of crap.

**Top Ten Cardio Machines**
1. StepMill
2. Treadmill
3. StairMaster
4. Rowing Machine
5. Stationary Bike
6. Elliptical
7. Arc Trainer
8. Trampoline Bullshit

9. Rock Climbing Wall
10. Fitness Flyer

## RUNNING TO THE DOCTOR

Around 3 million years ago, man began a form of terrestrial locomotion known as running in order to hunt animals over long distances and lengths of time. Fast-forward to the 16th century in England, and swordsmen began running as part of their training. The Irish soon followed, and in the 1960s, American Bill Bowerman traveled to New Zealand and then returned to the United States and wrote a book called *Jogging.* As boring as it sounds, this piece of literature began the "running craze" as millions of Americans hit the pavement in little shorts that should only be worn by a kickboxer in Thailand.

Without question, the most debilitating form of exercise today is running. Between 65 and 80 percent of runners will suffer an injury each year.[1] Some suffer from plantar fasciitis, others rupture their Achilles tendon, but the most common injury is to the knee joint. Plain and simple, if you're not hunting a wild boar in the jungle with a spear or bolting out of a bank toward a getaway car, you should not be running. Yet, two billion people worldwide destroy their knees daily as they pound the pavement, dirt, or treadmill for 4, 5, or even 10 miles. Take a look at somebody who has just finished a long run, and you'll witness the likes of a baby giraffe attempting to walk. If you enjoy running, limit the distance to three miles and no longer than 30 minutes. If you overdo it, the "runner's high" will end in agony in an orthopedic surgeon's waiting room.

Safer on the joints, and just as effective for your heart, walking on a treadmill at an incline for 30 to 40 minutes is my cardio of choice. I do 30 minutes at a speed of 4.0 MPH at a 5 percent incline. If you are just starting out, I recommend a speed of 3.5 MPH at a 5 percent incline for 30 minutes. With each step, squeeze your glutes and don't hold on to the rails.

# CHAPTER 11
# The Ultimate Antidepressant

**AN ANTIDEPRESSANT NAMED EXERCISE**

We all get depressed at times, and how can we not? We spend a third of our life working. That right there is enough to send even the Dalai Lama into a tailspin. Add on financial stress, family stress, and walking in on your girlfriend face down, ass up with your best friend in your own bed while she's ovulating, and you have every reason to feel a little bit down. The key is being able to get out from under that dark cloud and back into the sun. Enter exercise.

Lifting weights has always been my outlet to deal with a violent upbringing and being picked on in school. It has also helped me build confidence throughout my life. As a kid, when I felt alienated, depressed, and worthless, I would go to the gym and pump iron for hours to alleviate the pain. By controlling my body, I was able to compensate for my chaotic mind. It was

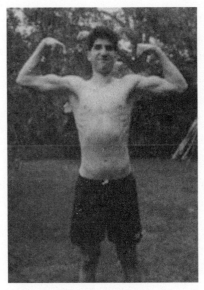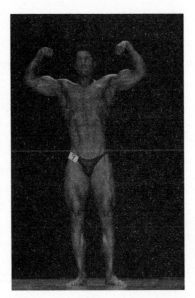

*A scrawny kid with big dreams.*

a form of character armor, and unlike with therapy, I could see tangible results. A bigger chest, a smaller waist—it was all visible right there in the mirror. No matter how bad of a day I am having, I always walk out of the gym feeling better than when I walked in. One explanation for this boost in mood are the chemical changes that take place during intense exercise such as increases in brain opioid levels and endocannabinoids, which can indirectly increase dopamine levels.[1] Serotonin, which is the hormone responsible for mood, sleep, and appetite, has also been proven to increase during weight lifting. The sense of accomplishment felt after completing a hard workout should also not be shortchanged and is incredibly valuable to your sense of self-worth. When we lift weights, we not only hoist up the iron gripped tightly in our palms, but we also exorcise the stress that weighs us down in daily life. With each repetition, anxiety is mollified, depression is diminished, and just like the weights, our mood is lifted. Metaphorically speaking, lifting weights is superior to all other forms of exercise. Running suggests fleeing from your problems, while spinning implies expending energy without getting anywhere. Lifting weights is an antidepressant, meditation, and an exploration of self. You challenge your body, train your mind, and expand your pain threshold. The intense focus and discipline is then applied to other areas of your life, and you set goals and work hard until you reach them.

Psychologically, having muscles is like walking down the street with a pitbull. At 6'3", 215 pounds, I am a poor choice to mug because it appears that if I get my hands on a criminal, I will hurt him. Thankfully, my lifetime record in fights is an astounding 0–0. That's right, not one fight, not even a scuffle. The opposite of militant, I view bodybuilding as an art project, except the body is the canvas, the weights are the paintbrush, and the food is the paint. Unlike a finished piece, the body is constantly changing, which is why daily exercise is so important to maintain order in both your mind and body. Whenever you feel down in the dumps, go to the gym and lift some weights. The worse you feel, the more you need it. I guarantee you'll leave the gym feeling a whole lot better.

## SETTING GOALS

I'm not going to ask you to walk across hot coal or tell you that the subconscious mind holds the secrets to the Universe. Tony Robbins already does that. I'm also not going to tell you that "You can do anything if you put your mind to it," because that's just plain bullshit. No matter how much I visualize and believe that I'm going to win a NBA slam dunk contest, it's never going to happen. Similarly, if you are a singer with no talent, an unwavering belief that you'll one day sell out Madison Square Garden is a recipe for disaster. That is why setting realistic fitness goals should be the first thing you do before you ever step on a treadmill. Honest self-evaluation must be implemented, or the only goal you'll consistently reach is disappointment. For example, if you are 50 pounds overweight, your short term goal could be to lose four pounds in one month but should not be to lose 40 pounds in two months. Sometimes it helps to go over goals with a close friend, family member, or trained professional in order to know what is overzealous and what is realistic.

And make sure you write them down! According to a study done by Gail Matthews at Dominican University, those who wrote down their goals and shared them with friends with weekly updates accomplished their goals on average 33 percent more than those that just formulated them.[2] So, grab a pen and start jotting down realistic goals. Lose 10 pounds in three months, gain five pounds of muscle in a year, run two miles without stopping, last a minute longer in bed, fit into your dress from prom night. Give yourself a clear objective and then create your plan of attack to achieve it. And when you reach that goal, cross it off the list, celebrate, and then create a new one. The late comedy legend, David Brenner, once told me that life is a series of "nexts." The next show, next meal, next workout, next set, next vacation, next marriage, next child, next pet, next parking ticket. It's about what's next! Keep moving forward and don't ever look back.

## MOTIVATION

Each person responds differently to criticism and is motivated by various stimuli. Some thrive on tough love such as being told by a doctor that if they don't lose weight, they'll have a heart attack and die. To others, fear makes them spiral even more.

According to humanistic psychologist Abraham Maslow, there are two kinds of motivation: deficiency motivation and growth motivation.[3] Deficiency motivation is when a person lacks something and is motivated to fix it. An overweight person needs to lose twenty pounds, so he begins working out five days a week and eating healthy foods and eventually loses the excess weight. Since the deficiency no longer exists, he loses all motivation and is content with his new body. That brings him back to his former sedentary lifestyle of TV and potato chips, and he gains all the weight back. Now, he has a deficiency once again, and it's time to hit the gym.

A much healthier form of motivation is growth motivation, in which the individual strives to improve no matter what. This type of motivation never ceases and is what Maslow described as the key to being "self-actualized" and reaching one's full potential.[3] There are so many benefits to being in great shape that motivation shouldn't come so difficult. You will have more energy and confidence, and live a higher quality of life. If standing in front of the mirror naked motivates you to work out, then by all means, strip down! If taping a picture to the fridge of a heavier version of yourself keeps you from eating that late night bowl of ice cream, then go for it. One of the joys of working out is that you can always improve and look better. In that, growth motivation comes easy. Here are a few ways to keep growth motivation in action:

- Visualize constantly how you wish to look and be specific and, more important, realistic given your body type. At 6'3", it would be silly for me to model myself after Sylvester Stallone, who is much shorter.

- Read books, magazines, and websites that have inspiring photos and great articles.
- Make sure you schedule your workout into your Google calendar and give it a time slot, as you would any meeting or doctor's appointment. It deserves to be a priority in your life.

## MASLOW THE GYM RAT

In 1943, humanistic psychologist Abraham Maslow proposed a theory of self-actualization in which he laid out a blueprint for one to follow in order to reach their full potential. He described a hierarchy of needs that every person must receive in order to maximize their life:

Physiological Needs: Food, water, air, shelter, clothing

Safety Needs: Personal and financial security, health and well-being

Love/Belonging: Family, friendship, and sex

Esteem: Confidence, achievement, and the respect of others

Self-Actualization: Full human potential realized and expressed through art, inventions, and accomplishment

On this list, virtually all of your needs can be met by going to the gym.

- You'll be sheltered, showered, and fed water. (Physiological)
- You'll look and feel strong. (Safety)
- You'll make new friends and sleep with some of them. (Love/Belonging)
- You'll build confidence through exercise and accomplish new feats of strength. (Esteem)

- You'll go home from the gym feeling like a champion and then paint a masterpiece and write a novel. (Self-Actualization)

Follow Maslow's advice and go to the gym.

## THE ROLE OF HEROES

Warren Buffett emulated Benjamin Graham, Pete Sampras shadowed Rod Laver, and I strived to build a body like Steve Reeves. Long before Arnold Schwarzenegger and Lou Ferrigno,

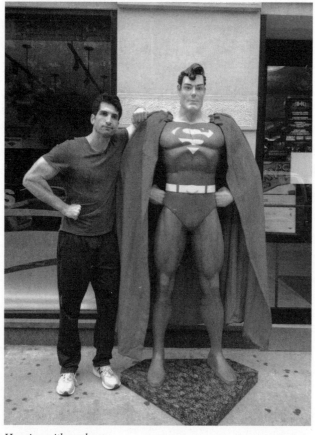

*Hanging with my hero.*

"The Natural" Steve Reeves was the original action hero and first to play Hercules on the big screen.

The boy from Montana made a fortune in Italy, becoming the king of "B" movies, and to this day, he is widely considered to have one of the best physiques of all time. His training was basic and his diet was clean. Rather than try to build a massive, bulky physique on his 6'1" frame, he strived for proportion and symmetry. Everything flowed from the top down, and he was one of the first bodybuilders to have a twenty-inch differential between his shoulders and his waist. He made the "V" torso famous and became an idol to virtually every bodybuilder to follow. In his prime, he won the Mr. America and Mr. Universe competitions at a weight of 215 pounds. By today's standards, he would appear a stick figure, as bodybuilders who are 5'6" now weigh that much. Still, he was ahead of his time and set the standard for aesthetics. I think it is important to have somebody to model yourself after. Now, I don't mean copy, as we all have to distinguish ourselves individually. However, it's good to take bits and pieces away from your idols. Just make sure you pick someone with a similar height and build.

## TRANSCENDENTAL MEDITATION

For my 21st birthday, my mother asked me what I wanted for a gift, and when I told her that I would like to learn Transcendental Meditation (TM), she was confused and concerned and questioned my motive. Itching to try stand-up comedy, I explained that many of my comedy heroes including Andy Kaufman, Jerry Seinfeld, and Howard Stern were all meditators who claimed that TM helped them manage stress and foster creativity. After accepting that her only son may be insane, she obliged and financed the education. It turned out to be one of the best gifts that I have ever received.

For three days, I went to my teacher Sheila's home in Newton, Massachusetts, where she educated me on Vedic science, gave me a mantra, and taught me how to meditate. Lower blood pressure, improved memory, and increased activity in the frontal and parietal cortices of the brain (the areas associated with creativity) were among the benefits found in over 340 studies. In the 1970s, Harvard physician, Dr. Herbert Benson researched TM and both wrote the book and coined the phrase "The Relaxation Response." He defined this as "A physical state of deep rest that changes the physical and emotional responses to stress, and the opposite of the fight or flight response."

The benefits of meditation on the body are vast and include reduced oxygen consumption, improved release of carbon dioxide, and lowered rates of respiration.[4] Transcendental meditation also raises your natural growth hormone level and lowers production of thyroid stimulating hormone (TSH), allowing for maximum bodybuilding results.[4]

As I began to meditate twice a day for twenty minutes as instructed, I noticed a deeper and deeper level of relaxation and found myself in a more focused, optimistic mood. According to the founder of TM, his holiness, Maharishi Mahesh Yogi, "Sitting quietly while meditating brings increased energy to daily life in the same way that pulling an arrow back six inches on a bow allows for the release of great energy when the arrow is shot forward." If you are looking to build your body, calm your mind, and lower your level of anxiety, you may want to give transcendental meditation a try. A lifelong skeptic, I have found TM to help considerably. Since I began meditating fifteen years ago, I am a much happier, calmer person, and my workouts are much more focused.

## SLEEP

To be completely honest, I'm having a lot of trouble with this section right now because I didn't sleep very well last night. Sadly, I'm far from alone. According to a 2011 poll conducted by the National Sleep Foundation, half of all adults admitted to rarely getting a good night's sleep. Personally, I average six hours of sleep a night and on that splendid, rare occasion that I get a full eight hours, I feel like a different person. I'm less irritable and more alert, and I might even help the homeless. Unfortunately, since I wake up at 5 a.m. to train clients starting at 6 a.m., to get eight hours of sleep would mean going to bed at 9 p.m., and unless you are a Buddhist monk or an eight-year-old, 9 p.m. is not a universally accepted bedtime.

When it comes to building muscle, a bad night of sleep is a catabolic catastrophe. In fact, the cleanest diet and most intense workout routine in the world will be offset if you do not get enough rest at night. When working out with weights, you break down muscle fibers that must recover and grow during deep sleep. And 30–45 minutes after falling asleep, human growth hormone (HGH) is released into the blood and is at its highest level two hours into sleep.[5] Having high levels of HGH in the blood allows the muscle to absorb amino acids at a high capacity and facilitate muscle growth.[5] When you don't get enough sleep at night, research has shown that the following evening you have higher levels of cortisol, a hormone release by the adrenal gland to deal with stress. Elevated levels of this hormone hinder the absorption of amino acids into the muscle cells and inhibit bone formation so that your body cannot grow and repair properly. High levels of cortisol also raise your blood pressure and increase appetite. To make matters worse, when you are sleep deprived, your fat cells release less leptin, a hormone that suppresses appetite.[5] So getting too little sleep not only destroys any chance of muscle growth, but it puts your body in the right hormonal balance to gain fat. Wow, a 9 p.m. bedtime is starting to sound better and better. Some helpful tips to improve your quality of sleep include:

- Set a 2 p.m. caffeine cutoff time to avoid later disruptions in sleep.
- Avoid artificial light before bed (television, laptops, cell phone).
- Never exercise right before bed and try to allow three hours after a workout before going to bed.
- Avoid alcohol at night.
- Finish eating dinner a few hours before going to bed to allow time for digestion.

## SEPARATE BEDROOMS

My wife and I have a wonderful marriage, and one of the secrets to our success is separate bedrooms. Not separate beds, separate bedrooms. When our friends learn this about us, they say "Wow, you guys are weird." Maybe, but we're also well rested. They say, "But there's nothing better than a warm body next to you in bed." Yes, there is, and it's called a cool mattress. Let's face it, having somebody else in bed with you can't help you sleep better, they can only wake you up. In fact, when my wife and I were first dating, I always found it peculiar that such a petite woman slept on a king-size bed. At 5'4", she sleeps diagonally and "starfishes" by flailing her arms out to the side, which makes another person next to her near impossible. In fact, it's not uncommon that she'll wake up completely horizontal across her mattress. A light sleeper who has suffered from insomnia most of her life married a man who is an absolute nightmare unconscious. I snore like a beast, kick, twitch, scream, and even laugh. Early on, we'd attempt unsuccessfully to spend the night together, and we'd both be miserable zombies the next day. When we decided to move in together, we made sure that we each had our own bedroom, and when we got married, we even considered putting in our wedding vows "I promise to love you for better, for worse, for richer, for poorer, in sickness and in health, in separate bedrooms until death do us part."

Thankfully, my wife's sleep has improved with the help of a sleep expert and several accessories that include a white noise machine, sleep mask, body pillow, mouthguard, and blackout curtains. Her sleep expert shares the popularly held belief that a bed is to be used for sleep and sex only. And as wonderful as watching TV in bed can be, the artificial light and association made by your brain can make falling asleep very difficult. She taught her that even reading in bed is unacceptable and if she can't sleep, move to a chair or couch before opening a book.

Back in the 1950s, it was not unusual for Grandma and Grandpa to have separate beds. They understood the importance of sleep and the annoyance of being woken up. We took it one step further and put ourselves in completely different rooms on opposite ends of the apartment. We did this because we love each other. If you're in a relationship and prefer your own bed or bedroom, you may insult your partner with the suggestion of sleeping separately. But don't worry, they'll get over it, and they may even agree to it. Here's hoping.

## My Ten Commandments for Tranquility

1. Elicit the "relaxation response" every day through either meditation, yoga, or visual imagery.
2. Happy wife, happy life. Be good to your partner.
3. Get as much sleep each night as possible.
4. Try not to get stressed out about that which you can't control.
5. Do not smoke or do drugs. Stay clear.
6. Praise more than you disparage.
7. Pay careful attention to negative speech and nip it in the bud.
8. Perform your job with energy and enthusiasm.
9. Learn to say "No."
10. Eat healthy, train hard, and act with love and humility.

# CHAPTER 12
# The Personal Trainer Manifesto

Gym members often hire personal trainers to combat the laziness inherent in the human spirit. A good personal trainer combines the qualities of a therapist, bartender, high school football coach, and loyal friend. Like any successful long-term relationship, trust is at the forefront. The client wants to be pushed but not knocked over. Goals must be set and reached or the wallets are withdrawn and shut.

Unfortunately, most trainers don't have a clue how to design a half-decent workout program. They get paid to be talking heads and instruct their client to warm up on a treadmill for twenty minutes only to move a pin on some useless machine for the remaining forty. The client pays an obscene price and gets a lackluster workout. In New York City, a large number of trainers are unemployed actors and models who ask themselves, "Should I be a trainer or a waiter?" I say, "Be a waiter! Please! Stay the fuck out of the gym and save your client the future as a hunchback."

In thousands of gyms across the country, I have noticed a growing trend of fat personal trainers. Not only is this hypocritical, it's downright inexplicable. Why would anyone waste their money on a fat personal trainer? That's like going to a suicidal life coach. If I had a fat trainer, I wouldn't believe one word he said. He'd be like, "Do ten push-ups!" I'd say, "It's not going to make me fat, is it?" A trainer needs to lead by example and earn that t-shirt that says "Master Trainer." They should look the part and think of it as an acting exercise. If you have to guess which one is the trainer and which is the client, there is something seriously wrong.

Lately, it seems as if there are more "celebrity trainers" than there are celebrities. Every day, a self-proclaimed "celebrity trainer" pops up with some new "groundbreaking" exercise routine that promises to change your body and, more important, strengthen your core! It's all about the core! It's working my core! Anyone remember when the core was known as the stomach, cardio meant jogging, and yoga was just some weird shit that hippies did? Now, I'm all for innovation and advancement, but the fitness wheel was built a long time ago by the ghosts of fitness past such as Jack LaLanne, Bill Pearl, and Steve Reeves. For decades, this wheel has been repackaged, repainted, and sold at some ridiculous price that millions of Americans are willing to purchase. Wow, the Ab Bench! I can just sit on my ass and work my abs! Then there's a new Perfect Pushup, because the old one wasn't good enough. The bottom line is that none of this is necessary. Simplicity works, and fads pass.

As a personal trainer, I often double as a therapist in my training sessions. Clients tell me things they won't tell their spouse, and it's my job to be discreet and offer as much support as possible. If I had to make a choice between a good trainer or a good therapist, I'd pick the trainer. Unlike talk therapy, where you sit on a couch and your progress is hidden, a client at the gym can see their pumped-up biceps, tight glutes, and shredded six-pack. This tangible evidence gives the client an instant lift that talk therapy cannot—and it does so at a third of the price!

## LESS TALKING, MORE TRAINING

Many people reading this have either had a trainer or worked out near a trainer who just wouldn't shut up. Loquacious and bombastic, the trainer compromises the workout with a cacophony of noise worse than any garage band. Whether the trainer describes his drunken weekend at the strip club, his new iPhone, or his girlfriend who he believes is cheating on him, the workout focuses on one person: himself. He is using his client's training session for his own psychoanalysis and getting paid for it! As P. T. Barnum said, "There's a sucker born every minute."

My client and dear friend, Frank Bruni, has a motto that he implemented early on when we first began working together many years ago. It goes, "Less talking, more training." Translation: Shut up and focus on the workout, a motto that has made me an infinitely better trainer. Trainers need to be reminded that their job is to help their client get in the best shape possible. Of course, you want to make the hour as entertaining as possible, but never at the expense of the workout. You must evaluate constantly whether the client is reaching their goals and if not, figure out why. Are they working out hard enough, or is it time to completely revamp the workout to shock their body? Is their diet a mess? Are they doing enough cardio? Is their trainer a talking head who needs to shut his mouth? These are all questions that need to constantly be asked and answered.

## COUNTING: AN ELUSIVE SKILL
A good trainer can help you get into great shape, but don't expect them to always count to twenty successfully. For some reason, over the course of an hour, we always screw up and make a mistake. Personally, I consistently skip the number six, and whether I miscalculate for demonic reasons, out of sheer boredom, or just the inability to count like a first grader, I may never know. What I do understand is that it really pisses off my clients. The vast majority become most livid when I undercount, while a few masochists prefer that to overcounting, thereby cheating them out of the most crucial reps of a set.

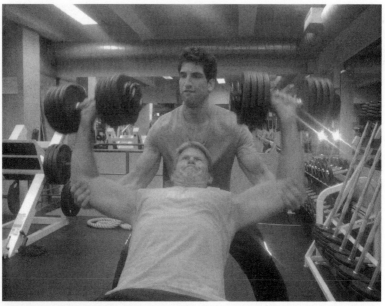

*Chuck blasts his chest while I count badly.*

Thankfully, we as trainers are not sought after for our intellect. History may reveal that there has never been a personal trainer who won Jeopardy, nor are there any Rhodes scholars currently serving as "weight caddies" at the local YMCA. If you hire a trainer, you should expect them to be punctual, knowledgeable, and attentive, but don't expect them to be able to count.

## THE MANY FACES OF TRAINER

If you're looking to hire a trainer, here are a few you should stay away from:

**The "Life Coach" Trainer:** Anyone who claims to be a "life coach" is more delusional than you will ever be. Life coaching can be traced back to the teachings of Benjamin Karter, a failed college football coach turned motivational speaker. With no formal training, they charge insane fees to provide a service that can be extremely destructive for the client.

**The iPhone Trainer:** This guy couldn't care less about training his client. Often in great shape, the iPhone trainer spends the hour texting, talking, and checking out the women working out around him. He often sits in one spot, yelling irrelevant instructions to a client in desperate need of a trainer.

**The New Age/Guru/Trainer:** She rambles on and on about energy, the alignment of planets, and her latest yoga retreat. She preaches about evolving and finds solace in her yogi/vegan lifestyle. Mercury is in retrograde, and she resides somewhere on Mars. For the last 30 minutes of the workout, she'll have you lie down with your eyes closed and meditate and then remind you to "Thank the Universe for all your gifts."

**The Model Trainer:** This guy's never seen a mirror he doesn't like and reminds himself constantly of his beauty while his client is squatting with a rounded spine. Your money is going toward his new headshots, not a better body. He cancels every other workout in order to make his cattle call audition for the new "Dr. Scholl's" print ad. He has his priorities straight, and they don't involve you.

## CLIENT GOALS

One of the biggest mistakes that trainers make is forgetting that the client is not them. Their goals are not your goals, nor should they be. Just because you want a six-pack and 20-inch arms does not mean that your client does. Therefore, you cannot always train them like you would train yourself. Too often, personal trainers go into autopilot mode and take client after client through the exact same workout. The 80-year-old man does the same routine as the 26-year-old woman who preceded him an hour before. Sometimes the workout even matches the one the trainer did himself earlier in the day. How's that for lazy? It is not uncommon to see a trainer focusing on chest and biceps exercises with a morbidly obese client. They don't need 24-inch biceps, they need fat loss. Step-ups, jump rope, squats, and even jumping jacks can help with fat loss. Just keep their whole body moving and their heart rate up.

Each client's workout should be unique to his or her goals, needs, and physical capabilities. If you sense that your trainer is phoning it in hour after hour with the same lame workout, it's probably time for a change.

## THE WORST TRAINER EVER

Charlatans exist in all walks of life, and they often go unexposed, spewing out verbal diarrhea to anyone who will listen. As the NYC antiterrorism adage dictates, "If you see something, say something." In my 12 years as a trainer, I have worked closely with hundreds of other trainers and have seen virtually everything in a gym—pro bodybuilders, contortionists, male strippers, and even an ex-con. To this day, I have never seen a worse one than the one who sadly has consistently taught his clients horrible form and bad eating habits, and replaced lack of knowledge with cheerleading. "Beautiful, you can do it, you're the best," can often be heard as his client strenuously lifts her water bottle to her lips with deep focus and proceeds to take a perfect swig with her knees bent, shoulders back, and eyes straight ahead.

He became a trainer like so many others by paying 400 dollars to take a certification exam that a chimp could pass. He knows one workout that involves the BOSU ball, a half-circle rubber apparatus that he must use for every exercise. For weeks, I would get to the gym early and hide that piece of equipment just so I could see him scramble when he realized that he had no "workout" to deliver. Was it juvenile on my part? Yes. Does this kind of trainer destroy the integrity of the gym and make trainers look bad? Yes. He conducts his scheme right there in the open and could easily be ignored and go unnoticed if it weren't for his unremitting voice that can only be described as auditory rape. Personally, I think that he should be arrested and charged with impersonating a trainer, also known as fraud. Here are the top 10 stupidest things I've ever heard the "Worst Trainer Ever" utter:

1. "Keep your eyes in your head, breathe through your neck, and focus on your belly button."
2. "The core is love and love is the core."
3. "Alignment is a gift to yourself."
4. "Think of your arms as branches and your legs as tree trunks."

5. "Focus on your ensemble muscles."
6. "Engage your lats." (while doing leg extensions)
7. "Come to my one-man show. It's going to be amazing."
8. "You don't sweat, you sparkle."
9. "Your posture is 5 percent better each week when we do this exercise."
10. "I love being a trainer."

## THE BEST TRAINER EVER

In my 20 years in the iron game, I have been influenced by such legends as Arnold Schwarzenegger, Lou Ferrigno, Frank Zane, and Steve Reeves. As I have grown older, the guy who I look up to the most is the late, great "Godfather of Fitness," Jack LaLanne, who, in my opinion, is the greatest ambassador of all time for fitness and helped millions of people around the world live a healthier lifestyle.

Clearly an obsessive personality, Jack LaLanne worked out two hours every day from 5 to 7 a.m. and claimed to have not eaten dessert in 40 years. He attributed all of his success to his supportive wife and truly practiced what he preached. Here are some of his beliefs and rules that he stuck to every single day of his life:[1]

1. A glass of wine every night at dinner. He chose either red or white zinfandel.
2. No processed foods. According to Jack, "If man made it, don't eat it. And if it tastes good, spit it out."
3. Heavy Fruit and Vegetable (Raw) Consumption. "I have at least 5 or 6 pieces of fresh fruit every day and 10 raw vegetables."
4. No Dairy. "It's not good for you. It's good for a suckling calf. Are you a suckling calf?"

5. Rely on Your Woman. "My wife is my protector. Without her, I'm nothing. Sure, she wants to please me, and I want to please her. We've been together over 53 years. She is my lover, my partner, my best friend."
6. Antiorganic Foods. "It's a bunch of bull."
7. No Debt/Own Outright. "When I started out, we were very poor. My dad would say, Kid, if you are going to buy something, pay with cash. Never get into debt with anything. I never forgot that. Anything that Elaine and I would do—we'd own it. No partners ever. I don't think about wealth."
8. Help People. "We both believe one thing: Wanting to help people who help themselves."
9. Exercise and Nutrition. "Exercise is king. Nutrition is queen. Put them together and you've got a kingdom!"
10. Anything is possible if you love what you do and work hard. "Billy Graham is about the hereafter. I'm for the here and now."

## ADVICE TO TRAINERS

As a trainer who has lived and breathed fitness since I was 12 years old, the best advice I ever received from another trainer was "If you go to bed dreading training someone the next day, don't train them." Like a relationship, when you work with someone who is really motivated, the results and experience can be wonderful and very fulfilling. Conversely, when the client is negative and unwilling to put in the effort, it's time to cut them loose.

## Training a Stinky Client

He was an older fellow in a gray tank top and arrived ten minutes early for our first ever training session. Let's call him Joe, okay? So, Joe and I shook hands, and I'm immediately struck by how bad Joe smells. I couldn't decide whether it was dirty gym clothes, no deodorant, or both. No, this was worse. Quite frankly, Joe smelled like a rotting dog. When I began the workout on the lat pulldown machine, I quickly realized my error, as Joe's arms extended up above his head, and his smell hit me like a ton of bricks. I was out on my feet for a standing eight count but was able to recover in time for the 15th and final rep. Realizing the bind I was in, I thought, *I got it! We won't do any exercises where he puts his arms above his head.* In other words, we would need to do lots of leg exercises. I also found that hammer curls and triceps kickbacks worked safely but to stay away from all shoulder and chest, exercises. I made him do crunches with his arms across his chest, and when he completed his third set of 25, I had survived. It was a great workout for both of us. Like a client with an injury, I was able to work around stinky.

Exercises that work for stinky:

Leg Press

Leg Extensions

Lunges

Leg curls

Barbell curls

Low cable row

Crunches (arms crossed on chest)

Triceps cable pushdowns

Hammer curls

# EXERCISE INDEX

**SHOULDER EXERCISES**
**Lateral Raises:** Standing with your feet shoulder-width apart, hold the dumbbells with your arms fully extended down by your side. With a slight bend in the elbows, raise both arms out to the sides until they are slightly above shoulder height. Hold for a second and then slowly bring the weights back down. This exercise can also be performed seated with your arms hanging out to your side.

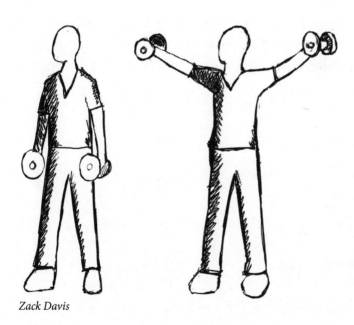

*Zack Davis*

**Barbell Upright Rows:** Holding a barbell in front of you with a palms-down, shoulder-width grip, raise the bar straight up to chest level, leading with your elbows. Slowly lower the bar.

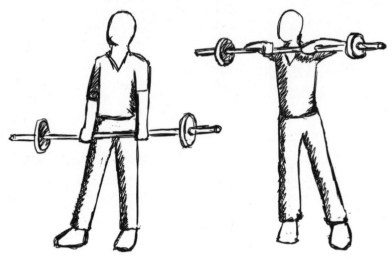

*Zack Davis*

**Bent-over Lateral Raises:** Seated on the edge of a bench, lean forward with dumbbells in each hand and elbows bent slightly. Lift the weights directly out to your side until your arms are

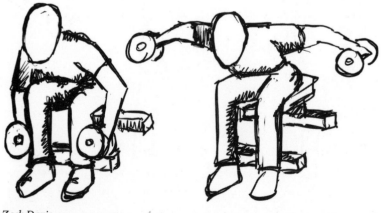

*Zack Davis*

level with your body. Squeeze your shoulder blades together and use a weight light enough that you can isolate this area (back of the shoulders/rear delts).

**Seated Dumbbell Press:** Seated on a bench with back support, lift dumbbells overhead in a triangle motion, coming together at the top. By dipping the elbows and stretching the shoulder, slowly lower the weights until they are at chin height and then press them back up just short of locking the elbows.

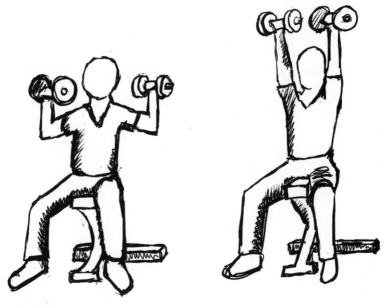

*Zack Davis*

## BICEPS EXERCISES
**Hammer Curls:** Standing with your feet-shoulder width apart, hold dumbbells at arm's length at your sides. With the palms of your hands facing each other and upper arms tight to your body, curl the dumbbells to shoulder level by bending the elbows and then slowly lower the weights back down. Do not

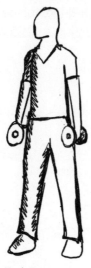
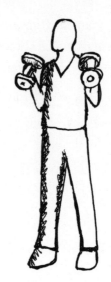

*Zack Davis*

snap or swing the weights up and make sure you contract the top of your forearms and your biceps.

**Barbell Curls:** Standing with your feet shoulder-width apart and knees bent, with a shoulder-width underhand grip, curl

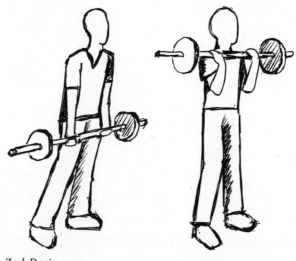

*Zack Davis*

the bar from your thighs up to your shoulders. At the top of the movement, make sure you contract the muscle; otherwise, it will just relax. Lower the weight back down slowly without fully locking the elbows.

## CHEST EXERCISES

**Incline Dumbbell Press:** Set a bench to a 30-degree incline. Press dumbbells above your chest until your elbows are nearly locked out. Lower the weights slowly down to chest level and then press the weight back up in a triangle motion until the dumbbells are almost touching above your chest. Lower again.

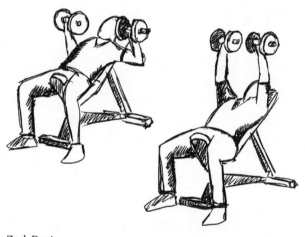

*Zack Davis*

**Bench Press:** Lying flat on a bench, grab the bar with a wider-than-shoulder-width grip and lift it off the rack with arms fully extended. Lower the weight to the bottom part of your chest, just short of touching. Press the weight back up, but do not lock out the elbows, as that takes tension out of the chest.

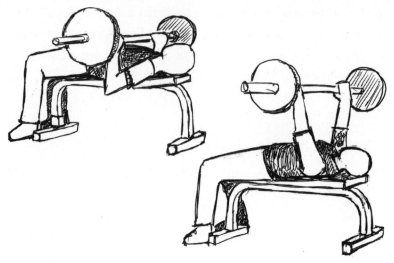

*Zack Davis*

Repeat the movement, stretching the chest at the bottom and contracting all the way up. When using a heavy weight, make sure you have a spotter present.

**Flat Dumbbell Flye:** Lying on a flat bench, press two dumbbells over your shoulders and bring them together at the top

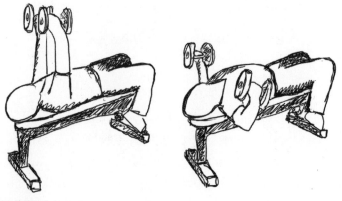

*Zack Davis*

with palms facing each other. With a slight bend in the elbows, slowly lower the weights in a semicircular motion until they are at chest level. Then press the dumbbells back up in the same arc, as if you're wrapping your arms around a tree trunk or giving a bear hug. Think of opening the chest on the negative (down) part of the motion and then closing the chest on the positive (up) part.

**Dips:** On a parallel bar, lift yourself up until your arms are straight. Slowly lower your body, leaning forward slightly until your elbows are at shoulder height. Do not go lower than this, as you will hurt your shoulder. Lift your body up until your arms are nearly straight (not fully) and then lower yourself down. Repeat as many times as you can and keep constant tension on the chest, shoulders, and triceps. Keep the same pace throughout the exercise.

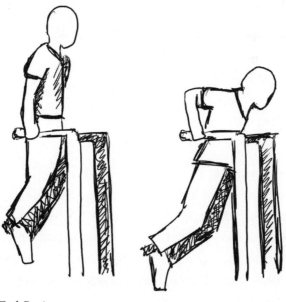

*Zack Davis*

## BACK EXERCISES

**Lat Pulldowns:** Sit on the chair of the lat pulldown machine with your knees secured under the pad. Set the pin to the appropriate weight and reach up to grab the bar with an overhand wide grip. With an arch in the back, pull the bar down to the top of your chest, focusing on pulling with your elbows and squeezing your shoulder blades together. Hold for a second at the bottom of the movement and then return it slowly to the starting position, all the while contracting and tensing the back muscles on the way up.

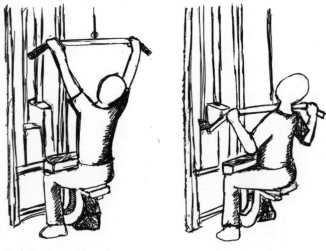

Zack Davis

**Pullovers:** Lying on a bench, hold one dumbbell directly over your chest with both hands by forming a triangle grip on the top part of the weight. With elbows slightly bent, slowly lower the weight back over your face and behind your head for a full stretch, letting in a big inhale as you do so, and then with a big exhale, using your rib cage, lift the weight back over your head until it's back over your chest.

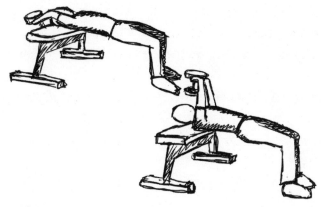

*Zack Davis*

**One-Arm Dumbbell Row:** With one knee up on a bench, lift the dumbbell with your opposite arm with your back arched and completely flat. Make sure to stick out your butt to maintain the proper arch in your back. Lift the weight up, thinking *pull with the elbow,* and squeeze your shoulder blade on the same side of your back. Lower the weight slowly and stretch out the entire back. After your last rep, switch legs on the bench and lift with the other arm.

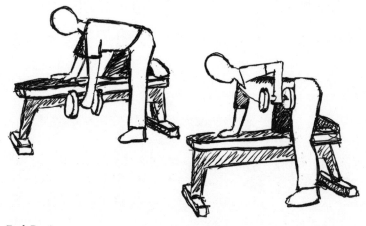

*Zack Davis*

**Pull-Ups:** Step up on a bench if you cannot reach the pull-up bar from the ground. With a wide overhand grip, pull your body up until your chest reaches the bar and then slowly lower your body to a full stretch. Pull yourself all the way up again and contract your shoulder blades together at the top of the movement.

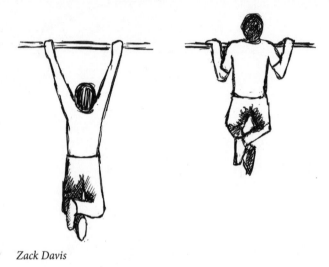

*Zack Davis*

**Deadlifts:** With your knees bent, butt low, and back arched, lift the bar off of the ground in a squat motion until you are

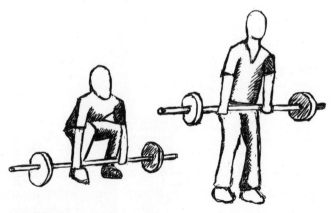

*Zack Davis*

standing fully erect. Pull your shoulders back slightly at the top of the movement and flex your back muscles. Lower the weight down in the same squat motion and repeat. You can also use a one hand over, one hand under grip if that is more comfortable.

**Bent Rows:** With an overhand grip just slightly wider than shoulder width, bend your knees, arch your back, and lift the barbell off of the ground. With your back completely flat, pull the weight up into your upper abdomen. Lower the weight just short of locking out your elbows and pull the weight back up. Pull with the elbows and contract the shoulder blades at the top of the movement.

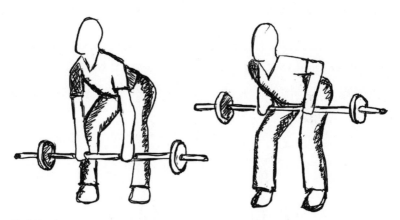

*Zack Davis*

## LEG EXERCISES
**Squats:** Step underneath a bar and rest it on your traps (the meaty part of the shoulder area). With a shoulder-width stance and toes pointed slightly out, bend your knees to squat down until your upper legs are parallel to the floor. Make sure your

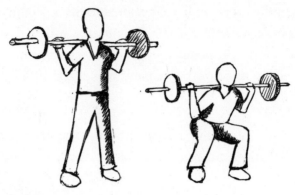

*Zack Davis*

back stays straight throughout the movement and think of sitting straight down into a chair. Using your quadriceps and hamstrings, lift your body back up straight to a standing position and then repeat the movement.

**Lunges:** Standing with dumbbells at arm's length, step forward with your right foot, allowing your body to drop as you bring the knee of your rear leg close to the floor. Push off with your

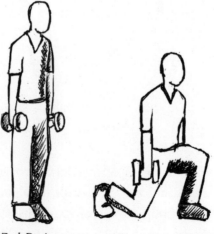

*Zack Davis*

front leg and return to the starting position. Do 12- 15 reps on the right leg locked in this position and then switch legs. Make sure your front knee never bends past your toes.

**Stiff-Legged Deadlifts:** Holding a barbell in front of you, lower the bar to the top of your feet. Bend your knees slightly during the descent and keep your waist straight, flexing only at the bottom. With your knees bent, lift the bar by extending at the hips until standing upright. Pull your shoulders back slightly if rounded.

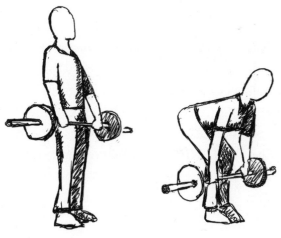

*Zack Davis*

## TRICEPS EXERCISES
**Triceps Cable Pushdowns:** Stand at a cable apparatus with the pulley in the top position. Using either a rope or v-handle, pull the attachment to a position at chest level and, with a shoulder-width stance with knees slightly bent, keep your upper arms tight to your torso and press the handle down until your arms are straight. Contract the triceps as hard as you can and then slowly return the attachment to chest level.

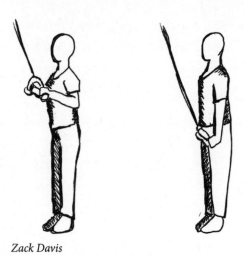

*Zack Davis*

**Lying Triceps Extensions (Skull Crushers):** Lying flat on a bench with feet on the floor, press an EZ bar overhead above your shoulders. Bend your elbows and slowly lower the bar to a position just past your forehead by your hairline. Now, press the weight up and back and straighten your arms, contracting the triceps and keeping the elbows pointed up and as still as possible. Slowly lower the weight back down and continue the movement. When using heavy weights, make sure you have a spotter.

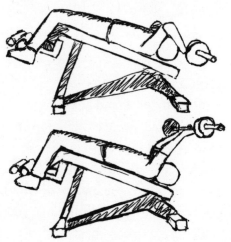

*Zack Davis*

**Dumbbell Kickback:** With one knee up on a bench, bend over and, with your elbow bent at shoulder height, kick back the weight until your arm is completely straight.

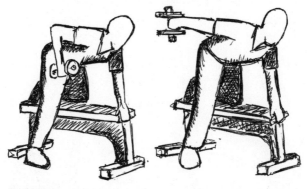

*Zack Davis*

## AB EXERCISES

**Leg Raises:** Lie on a flat bench with your butt placed at the bottom edge. Keeping your legs straight, feet together, and your lower back on the bench, raise your legs straight up until they're perpendicular to your body. Then, lower your legs below the level of the bench. Exhale as the legs come up, inhale as they go down.

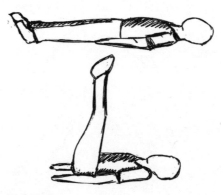

*Zack Davis*

**Knee-ins:** Sitting upright on the bottom of a bench, grab the bench at your sides and pull your knees into your body and your upper body into your knees. Think of it as an accordion and blow all the air out when the knees come in.

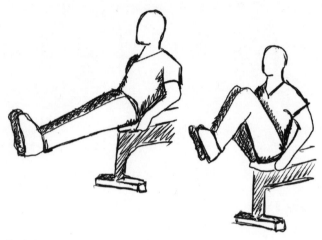

*Zack Davis*

**Crunches:** Lying on the floor, preferably a mat, put your legs up on a bench. Now, place your hands behind your head or fingers

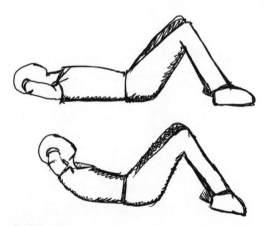

*Zack Davis*

behind your ears (harder) and crunch straight up toward the ceiling. Exhale at the top and then come down slowly without letting your head touch the ground.

**Cable Reverse Crunches:** Wearing ankle straps, attach both legs to a low pulley and lie flat on a mat with your hands halfway under your butt. Using a light weight, bring your knees into your chest and exhale at the top on the movement and then bring the legs back to full extension. Repeat this movement. This is a great exercise to build those deep ridges in the abs.

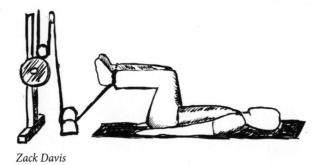

*Zack Davis*

# EPILOGUE

Obviously, there is much more to life than muscles, but there may be more life to live with them. As you get older and move into your golden years, the name of the game is *Don't Fall.* According to the National Council on Aging, falls are the leading cause of fatal and nonfatal injuries for older Americans.[1] The more muscle you have, especially on the lower body, the more stable you will feel and the better your balance will be. The problem is that each decade after age 30, you can lose 3–5 percent of your muscle mass if you eat poorly and don't exercise.[2] The less muscle you have, the more likely you are to fall, and, equally critical, the greater your fear of falling will be. This fear keeps seniors from being active in daily life. Through consistent strength training, stretching, and taking walks, seniors can retain their muscle and flexibility, and have the endurance to chase their grandchildren around the yard when they steal their toupee and hide it deep in the shrubs.

For the young whippersnappers who do not exercise, yet walk the Earth with boundless energy and an aura of invincibility, please know that the end is near. After age 25, your metabolic rate slows down by about 2 percent each decade.[3] That means that if you continue to do nothing but play video games, eat Pringles, and drink Mountain Dew, you will be obese and sick in no time. According to the Center for Disease Control, the leading cause of death in this country is heart disease.[4] Out of the 370,000 people who die annually from coronary heart disease, 200,000 of these deaths are preventable with changes in lifestyle.[5] Don't wait for Father Time to catch up to you. Get out in front of the storm and ride the wave of health as long as possible.

If quality and length of life are not enough to motivate you to lift weights, then pump iron for the attention and compliments that your new physique will garner. You can show off your body with daily pictures on Instagram, videos on Facebook, and motivational quotes like "Hard work beats talent but when talent works hard, it's over" on Twitter. Soothe your insecurities and fill that narcissistic void that keeps you standing in front of your parents' bathroom mirror with your iPhone, taking shots of your shredded six-pack for anyone who cares. If this has motivated you to hit the gym, I highly recommend talk therapy and a sabbatical from social media.

Like flossing, exercise needs to be performed daily for the rest of your life. While a great workout can be completed in under an hour, healthy eating must endure an entire day. The average person sleeps seven to eight hours a night, which makes eating a 16-to-17-hours-a-day job. That length of time provides a plethora of chances to open the refrigerator, pantry, or freezer and eat or drink something that will taste great and add fat to your body. Exercise, by comparison, is easy. You lift weights, run a few miles, or ride your bike through the park, and the muscles have been worked sufficiently. Over the years, I've had clients complain about not losing weight. I'd tell them, "Listen, I train you two hours a week, which leaves you 166 hours to fuck it all up."

No matter your age, sex, height, weight, or favorite football team—lifting weights should be the focal point of your workout routine. Around the weight routines, factor in flexibility training through stretching, yoga, and pilates. In addition, make sure to do some cardiovascular training to keep your heart in good health. Remember, consistency is the key to fitness. If you eat the right foods and train with intensity, you will never need to diet ever again.

# ACKNOWLEDGMENTS

Thank you to my wife, Rachel, for all your love and support.

Special thanks to Phil Hernon, Ed Connors, Ali Malla, and Patrick Malone, for your guidance and insight.

Thank you to my agent at Lotus Lane Literary, Priya Doraswamy, for your hard work and for believing in me. Thank you to Skyhorse Publishing and my editor, Julie Ganz, for your hard work and creativity.

Thank you to all my clients for putting your trust in me and filling my day with joy.

Finally, thank you to my family for instilling in me a passion for fitness.

# ENDNOTES

**CHAPTER 1**

1. Nordqvist, Christian. "Overcoming Leptin Resistance In The Battle Against Obesity." *Medical News Today*. N.p., 8 July 2015. http://www.medicalnewstoday.com/articles/251429.php

2. Wells, Jane. "Is "Organic" Really Organic? A Deep Dive into the Dirt." November 4, 2015. http://www.cnbc.com/2015/11/04/is-organic-really-organic-a-deep-dive-into-the-dirt.html.

3. Miller, Henry I. "The Colossal Hoax of Organic Agriculture." *Forbes*. July 29, 2015

4. TechSci Research. "Global Organic Food Market Forecast and Opportunities, 2020." August 2015. www.techsciresearch.com.

5. Bee, Peta. "Giving up bread can make you fat: Gluten IS good for you." *Daily Mail*. May 18, 2010.

6. De Nike, Lisa. "Crocodile and Hippopotamus Served as 'Brain Food' for Early Human Ancestors." John Hopkins University. N.p., 9 June 2010. Web.

7. Freedman, Rory, and Kim Barnouin. *Skinny Bitch*. Philadelphia: Running Press, 2005. Print. p 52.

8. Fox, Maggie. "Calcium From Supplements or Dairy Doesn't Strengthen Bones, Study Finds." NBCNEWS.com. N.p., 30 Sept. 2015. Web.

9. "7 Things That Happen When You Stop Eating Dairy." Prevention.com. N.p., 22 Sept. 2015. Web.

## CHAPTER 2

1. Brown, Brene. *Daring Greatly*. N.p.: Avery, 2012. Print.
2. Lambert, Craig. "The Way We Eat Now." *Harvard Magazine*. May-June 2004. http://harvardmagazine.com/2004/05/the-way-we-eat-now.html
3. Ferdman, Roberto A. "The Slow Death of the Home-cooked Meal." *Washington Post*. N.p., 5 Mar. 2015. Web.
4. Ingraham, Christopher. "The Average American Woman Now Weighs as Much as the Average 1960's Man." *Washington Post*. N.p., 12 June 2015. Web.
5. Pollan, Michael. "Out of the Kitchen, Onto the Couch." *New York Times Magazine*. N.p., 29 July 2009. Web.
6. Paul, Maria. "Religious Young Adults Become Obese By Middle Age." Northwestern.edu. N.p., 23 Mar. 2011. Web.

## CHAPTER 3

1. Donahoo, WT, J. A. Levine, and E. L. Melanson. "Variability in Energy Expenditure and Its Components." Current Opinion in Clinical Nutrition & Metabolic Care (2007): 599-605. Web.
2. Jones, Madeline. "Article Placeholder PLUS SIZE BODIES, WHAT IS WRONG WITH THEM ANYWAY?" Plusmodel-mag.com. N.p., 8 Jan. 2012. Web.
3. Nordqvist, Christian. "Eating Disorders Psychology/Psychiatry Mental Health Women's Health/Gynecology Eating Disorders Among Fashion Models Rising." Medical News Today. N.p., 8 July 2007. Web.
4. Dreisbach, Shaun. "Shocking Body-Image News: 97% of Women Will Be Cruel to Their Bodies Today." Glamour. com. N.p., 2 Feb. 2011. Web.
5. "Obesity and Overweight." Center for Disease Control and Prevention (cdc.gov). N.p., 13 June 2016. Web.

6. Kolata, Gina. "After The Biggest Loser, Their Body Fought to Regain Weight." *New York Times*. N.p., 2 May 2016. Web.

7. "Eating Disorder Statistics." South Carolina Department of Health. 2006. http://www.state.sc.us/dmh/anorexia/statistics.htm.

8. Pidd, Helen. "Skinny Male Mannequins Raise Eating Disorder Fears." The Guardian. 5 May 2010. www.theguardian.com/lifeandstyle/2010/may/05/skinny-male-mannequins-eating-disorder.

9. Boodman, Sandra G. "Eating Disorders: Not Just for Women." *Washington Post*. 13 March, 2007. http://www.washingtonpost.com/wp-dyn/content/article/2007/03/09/AR2007030901870.html.

10. Lukac, Michael. "Michael Jackson Autopsy Shows He Weighed 112 Pounds, Had Broken Ribs: Report." 28 June, 2009. http://www.ibtimes.com/michael-jackson-autopsy-shows-he-weighed-112-pounds-had-broken-ribs-report-286578.

11. Jaret, Peter. "Low Testosterone: Is Low T a Real Problem or Ad-Driven Fad?" AARP Bulletin. July/August 2014. http://www.aarp.org/health/conditions-treatments/info-2014/low-testosterone-therapy-controversy.html.

12. Alzado, Lyle. "I'm Sick and I'm Scared." *Sports Illustrated*. 8 July 1991. http://www.si.com/vault/1991/07/08/124507/im-sick-and-im-scared-the-author-a-former-nfl-star-has-a-dread-disease-that-he-blames-on-his-use-of-performance-enhancing-drugs%5D.

## CHAPTER 4

1. Szabo, A., A. Small, and M. Leigh. "The effects of slow- and fast-rhythm classical music on progressive cycling to

voluntary physical exhaustion." *Journal of Sports Medicine and Physical Fitness* 3, no. 39 (September 1999): 220-25.

2. Hutchinson, Alex. "How a Fitbit May Make You a Bit Fit." *New York Times.* 19 March 2016.

## CHAPTER 5

1. Dube, Rebecca. "No Puke, No Pain—No Gain." *Globe and Mail.* N.p., 11 Jan. 2008. Web.

2. Kroll, David. "Why Do Healthy People Die Running Marathons?" Forbes.com. N.p., 15 Apr. 2014. Web.

3. Goyanes, Cristina. "The Real Risk of Heart Attack During Endurance Exercise." Shape.com. N.p., n.d. Web.

4. Reynolds, Gretchen. "Ask Well: How Many Miles a Week Should I Run?" *New York Times.* N.p., 27 Nov. 2015. Web.

5. Sobel Fitts, Alexis. "Revisiting the Triathlon Death Rate." www.undark.org. N.p., 14 July 2016. Web.

6. Khan, Natasha, and Shannon Pettypiece. "Men Over 40 Should Think Twice Before Running Triathlons." Bloomberg.com. N.p., 21 June 2013. Web.

## CHAPTER 6

1. Wallace, Kelly. "Teens Spend a 'mind-boggling' 9 Hours a Day Using Media, Report Says." CNN.com. 3 November 2015. http://www.cnn.com/2015/11/03/health/teens-tweens-media-screen-use-report/

2. Stewart, James B. "Facebook Has 50 Minutes of Your Time Each Day. It Wants More." *New York Times.* 5 May 2016.

3. Schuenke, MD, J. M. McBride, and R. P. Mikat. "Effect of an Acute Period of Resistance Exercise on Excess Post-exercise Oxygen Consumption: Implications for Body Mass

Management." *European Journal of Applied Physiology* 86.5 (2002): 411-17. Web.

4. Goleman, Daniel. "Aggression in Men: Hormone Levels Are a Key." *New York Times.* N.p., 17 July 1990. Web.

**CHAPTER 7**

1. Raloff, Janet. "Reevaluating Eggs' Cholesterol Risks." Sciencenews.org. N.p., 2 May 2006. Web.

2. Neporent, Liz. "Bowl of Oatmeal a Day May Be Key to a Longer Life, Major Study Finds." abcnews.com. N.p., 6 January 2015. Web.

3. "Sweet Potato Offers Biggest Nutritional Gain for Your Buck." UPI. N.p., 14 March 2014. Web.

4. Rogers, Bridget. "Health Benefits of Eating Avocado— Can Avocados Cure Cancer?" Gazettereview.com. N.p., 30 January 2016. Web.

5. Rashidkhani, B., P. Lindblad, and A. Wolk. "Fruits, Vegetables and Risk of Renal Cell Carcinoma: A Prospective Study of Swedish Women." *International Journal of Cancer.* 3rd ser. 113 (2005): 451-55. Web.

6. Sterbenz, Christina. "The Entire 'Popeye' Franchise Is Based On Bad Science." Businessinsider.com. N.p., 17 January 2014. Web.

7. Kunkle, Frederick. "Walnuts Appear to Delay Onset of Alzheimer's Disease, New Study Finds." *Washington Post.* N.p., 21 Oct. 2014. Web.

8. Platkin, Charles. "The Diet Detective: You're Probably Drinking Enough Water." *Star-Telegram.* N.p., 11 September 2015. Web.

9. Stossel, John. "Is Bottled Water Better Than Tap?" Abcnews. com. N.p., 6 May 2005. Web.

10. "What Is It about Coffee?" *Harvard Health Publications.* N.p., January 2012. Web.
11. Abrams, Lindsay. "The Case For Drinking As Much Coffee As You Want." *The Atlantic.* 30 Nov. 2012: n. pag. Print.
12. O'Connor, Anahad. "Spike in Harm to Liver is Tied to Dietary Aids." *New York Times.* 21 December 2013

### CHAPTER 8

1. Brinkworth, Grant D., Jonathan D. Buckley, Manny Noakes, Peter Clifton, and Carlene Wilson. "Long-term Effects of a Very Low-Carbohydrate Diet and a Low-Fat Diet on Mood and Cognitive Function." *JAMA Internal Medicine* 169.20 (2009): n. pag. Web.
2. Fan, Shelly. "The Fat-fueled Brain: Unnatural or Advantageous?" *Scientific American* (2013): n. pag. Web.
3. Fedders, Aleisha K., "How Much Protein Do You Really Need?" *US News,* December 11, 2015. http://health.usnews.com/health-news/health-wellness/articles/2015/12/11/how-much-protein-do-you-really-need

### CHAPTER 9

1. Yu, Christine. "No Pain, No Gain? 5 Myths About Muscle Soreness." Daily Burn. July 17, 2014. http://dailyburn.com/life/fitness/doms-muscle-soreness/.
2. Cardore, Eduardo Lusa, Mikel Izquiedo, and Mariah Dos Santos. "Hormonal Responses to Concurrent Strength and Endurance Training with Different Exercise Orders." *The Journal of Strength and Conditioning Research* 26, no. 12 (December 2012): 3281-288. https://www.researchgate.net/publication/221726727_Hormonal_Responses_to_

Concurrent_Strength_and_Endurance_Training_with_
Different_Exercise_Orders.

3. Loh, Kep Kee, and Kanai, Ryota. "Higher media multi-task-ing activity is associated with smaller gray-matter density in the anterior cingulate cortex." September 24, (2014) PLOS ONE.

**CHAPTER 10**

1. Lobby, Mackenzie. "Avoid a Running Injury With the 10 Percent Rule." Active.com. http:/www.active.com/running/articles/avoid-a-running-injury-with-the-10-percent-rule.

**CHAPTER 11**

1. Linden, David. "Exercise, Pleasure, and the Brain." *Psychology Today.* N.p., 21 April 2011. Web.

2. Feinstein, Ashley. "Why You Should Be Writing Down Your Goals." *Forbes.* N.p., 8 Apr. 2014. Web.

3. Maslow, Abraham. *Toward a Psychology of Being.* 3rd Edition, Wiley, 1998.

4. Zane, Frank. *Fabulously Fit Forever.* Palm Springs: Zananda, 1993. Print.

5. Bennington, Vanessa. "How Sleep Deprivation Fries Your Hormones, Your Immune System, and Your Brain." Breakingmuscle.com. https://breakingmuscle.com/health-medicine/how-sleep-deprivation-fries-your-hormones-your-immune-system-and-your-brain.

**CHAPTER 12**

1. "Jack LaLanne's 29 Simple Rules For Life, Health and Fitness." Rippeder.com. http://rippeder.com/content/jack-lalannes-29-simple-rules-life-health-and-fitness.

## EPILOGUE

1. Fall Prevention Facts. National Council on Aging. 2017. https://www.ncoa.org/news/resources-for-reporters/get-the-facts/falls-prevention-facts/.
2. Boston, Gabriella. "Basal metabolic rate changes as you age." *Washington Post*, 5 March 2013. https://www.washingtonpost.com/lifestyle/wellness/basal-metabolic-rate-changes-as-you-age/2013/03/05/d26b1c18-80f1-11e2-a350-49866afab584_story.html?utm_term=.d2f846662c82.
3. Axe, Josh. "Sarcopenia: 10 Keys to Keep Your Muscle Mass Up as You Age." Dr Axe. - Food is Medicine. https://draxe.com/sarcopenia/
4. CDC. "Leading Causes of Death." Center for Disease Control and Prevention. 2015. https://www.cdc.gov/nchs/fastats/leading-causes-of-death.htm.
5. Jaslow, Ryan. "CDC: 200,000 heart disease deaths could be prevented each year." CBS News. 3 September 2013. http://www.cbsnews.com/news/cdc-200000-heart-disease-deaths-could-be-prevented-each-year/.